BENEATH CONTEMPT

ALSO BY HARRY COLFER

The Jono Series

Dead Regular

The Ambo Tales From The Frontline Series

Number 01: Abdominal Pain / Number 02: Allergy

Number 03: Animal Bite / Number 04: Assault

Number 05: Back Pain / Number 06: Breathing Problems

Number 08: Carbon Monoxide / Number 09: Cardiac Arrest

Number 10: Chest Pain / Number 11: Choking

Number 12: Convulsions / Number 13: Diabetic Problem

Number 15: Electrocution / Number 16: Eye Problem

Number 17: Fall / Number 21: Haemorrhage

Number 23: Overdose / Number 24: Pregnancy

Number 25: Psychiatric / Number 29: Traffic Accident

Number 31: Unconscious / Number 32: Unknown Problem

And

Collection 1: The First Twelve Tales

Collection 2: The Next Ten Tales

BENEATH CONTEMPT

HARRY COLFER

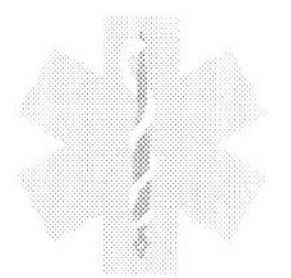

Beneath Contempt

Published by Harry Colfer Books

ISBN: 978-0-6489735-9-1 (Paperback Edition)

ISBN: 978-0-6489735-8-4 (eBook Edition)

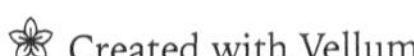

DISCLAIMER

This story is set on Mornington Island and takes place in 2013. Although the described medical procedures and techniques are authentic for that year and references are made to some real places and organisations, it is a work of fiction created for entertainment purposes only.

The paramedic characters portrayed in this story work for the Brisbane City Ambulance Service (B-CAS), which does not exist and is in no way meant to portray, or depict any existing, or former ambulance service, or organisation. The names, characters, or incidents mentioned herein are also completely fictitious. Any similarity to the name, character, or history of any person is entirely coincidental and unintentional.

To Julia

Your belief in me as well as your advice, assistance, tolerance, and support is what completes me and keeps me writing.

Love you and thank you.

1

AMBER NECTAR

I gazed at a bead of condensation as it formed on my glass, like sweat on the forehead of a dying man. Moonlight sparkled off its curved border, as it grew in size, gaining weight. Eventually, it overpowered its inertia and began trickling down the smooth surface, picking up momentum by consuming other droplets. As I watched, it occurred to me that the drop was a metaphor for life. We spend so much energy rushing about meeting others, but for what purpose? In the end, every individual just fades away, like the drop now lost within the ring of water around the bottom of my drink.

I reached out and picked up the tumbler on my second attempt, tipping it back to drain all the rum, the ice from my thermos long having melted. The liquid burned my throat as I swallowed and I stared at the glowing full moon through the distorted lens formed by the thick base of my glass.

It didn't seem to matter what shit happened in your life. The moon. The stars. The world. They all just carried on as they'd been doing for countless millennia. I slammed the glass down almost missing the little rickety camping table next to my deck chair and toppled over my bottle of Bundaberg Rum.

"Aahshit."

I lurched forward, grabbing for the bottle by my feet, but was relieved to discover I'd had the foresight to replace the cap. Refilling my glass, I snatched up the new measure and held it up to the star-scattered sky, toasting the moon. "Here's to life just carryin' on, ya heartless bastard."

I threw back the drink, but this time kept it in my mouth for a while, bathing my tongue in the velvet liquid. Parting my lips, I sucked the warm night air over the rum so my lungs received an intoxicating hit from the evaporated alcohol. I then swallowed it down and went to refill my glass when I noticed the silver-edged silhouette of a figure, standing on the beach near the dark water's edge.

It was a woman in her early thirties with long black hair, wearing a light flowing dress that billowed around her shapely legs in the gentle sea breeze. As she approached, I could see the sad look in her eyes that marred her beauty and I knew her bare feet would leave no footprints in the sand. I knew because I'd looked so many times before. I sighed and poured myself another drink.

"I's wondering when you'd show up. Glad yous could join me for our annivers'ry."

She came closer and stood about a metre or so away from me with her arms folded. I could almost touch her, smell her perfume. Despite the darkness, I could see every detail of her face, all the features I loved so much. The woman before me was Amber Shaw.

She shook her head with pity and smiled at me. "You need to stop your drinking, Jon."

"Ha." I took a swig from my tumbler. "Now ain't that the truth."

I dared not take my eyes away from her or even blink, in case reality returned and she disappeared, leaving me alone again.

"You know my shrink says you're just an hallooshination. A mental construct to help me cope with my post-traumatic stresh."

"And what do you think, Jon?"

I smiled and raised my glass. "I thinks I drink to catch another glimpse of you. I drink to pretend that you're real again. Jusht for a while. You see, I miss you so much. I'm lost..."

Tears streamed down my face, but I kept my eyes open so I wouldn't lose her again. She leant forward and kissed my wet cheeks, stroking my head before straightening up.

"I will always be with you, Jon. We had something special. But you need to move on. You've spent too long wallowing in self-pity and being here in this place isn't helping. You've got too much time to think."

She looked back at the waves rolling in and then at the sparse vegetation, as a gust of wind caused her hair to fly around. "You must leave this island and return to Brisbane. Restart your life and face your demons. And what's more, you need to do it now."

I laughed, but there was no humour in the sound. "Jusht my luck to get counselled by my own mental construct. How warped is that?"

I reached for another drink, but she snatched the bottle from my grasp. "I think you've had enough. What you need, Jon, is a wake-up call."

With that, she swung the bottle into the side of my head causing pain to explode throughout my skull. A new constellation appeared across my vision and the last thing I saw before I blacked out was Amber throwing the bottle into the sea.

Consciousness returned to me wielding a sledgehammer as I opened my right eye a fraction. I was lying on a combination of rock and sand on the upper part of the beach, looking out at the water lapping the shore. But the weak morning sun was too much for my optic nerve and the light forced me to retreat inside my skull. Despite the unforgiving mattress, I tried to go back to sleep, but someone kicked the sole of my boot.

"C'mon Jono. Up ya get, rise and shine. Looks like you fell out your deck chair last night and belted your head, eh. Hope you don't need patchin' up, seein' as you're on shift at twelve. You know the island needs you and I'm sure you don't want Albert treating you, eh."

I pushed myself up into a sitting position and rubbed my face, but instantly regretted it. A mixture of sand and congealed blood encrusted my right temple and I winced as I made a fingertip exploration of my newfound injury. I attempted to speak, but it felt like a roo had taken a crap in my mouth.

Screwing up my face, I squinted at the man whose tall lean body blotted out the rising sun, but the image was still too bright and I had to look away. Nevertheless, I knew who'd delivered my wake-up call. "What time's it, Charlie?"

"Time you were gettin' up for work, eh. I can't keep draggin' your sorry arse back to town every time you start your run of shifts."

He squatted down in front of me with amusement playing on his dark-skinned face and he rubbed his broad nose as if to conceal a smile. "I knew I'd find you here, my friend. You were seen leavin' town with your table and chair, eh."

"Well, aren't you the tracker?"

"Ha. Thought I'd get you this time, but what a surprise - you stink of booze, but no sign of a bottle. How d'you do it, Jono? One of these days I'm gonna catch you and you'll be up for a big fine, eh. You know Mornington's a dry island."

"Can't you give a guy a break. I think someone assaulted me."

He laughed. It was a warm sound that echoed from deep inside his belly. With a flick of his hand, he knocked his wide-brimmed Akubra to the back of his head and scratched the exposed wavy black hair. "Assaulted, out here? The only thing that assaulted you was gravity, eh. That and about four million mozzies. You look like you've come down with the measles. I'm surprised they didn't drink you dry, eh."

He looked out at the flat calm waters of the bay. Our two figures cast long shadows down the beach in the morning's golden glow. "Mind you, you're lucky a croc didn't drag you off. You must have a death wish sleepin' rough out here, eh."

"I just came to watch the sunset, didn't intend to stay the night."

"You never do. Now, get your butt in my car, so I can drive you back to your digs, eh. You need to clean yourself up before anyone sees you. You're a smart man, Jono. Why d'you insist on being so dumb?"

"It's a talent I have."

He stood and held out his hand to pull me up and I accepted the offer, although being upright seemed to invigorate the sadist with the sledgehammer. Charlie chuckled on seeing my face and then folded up my table and chair, throwing them into the tray of his marked-up dual cab police ute.

I climbed into the passenger seat and used the vanity mirror on the sun visor to check out my head. It was a small laceration that looked more from a rock than a bottle. Alcohol often caused my dreams to merge with reality.

Charlie swung himself in beside me. "You'll live, more's the pity. If we lose you, they may have to send us a real ambo, eh."

He started the engine and negotiated his way off the beach before bumping back along the dirt track towards the island's only town, Gununa. As the dust swirled up behind his car, he chuckled to himself. "How long does it take you to walk out here with that table and chair? It must be ten Ks or more."

"'Bout two hours. It can be relaxing."

"Ever thought of gettin' yourself a pushie?"

I tensed at the mere suggestion. I hadn't used a pushbike for about a year, ever since that night.

"You OK? You look like you've seen a ghost, eh."

"You don't know the half of it. No, mate, I'm OK. Just one of my flashbacks."

He glanced over at me, then stared at the road ahead. "You know, Jono, you were really fucked over last year, eh. You've got every right to be screwed up, but you'll get through it. I know you will, eh. Just hang on in there, mate."

I sighed. "Thanks, Charlie. And thanks for coming out to get me. I owe you one."

"What, another? Guess you're lucky I'm not countin', eh."

He flashed me a wide grin and we continued in silence for the rest of the trip. We soon pulled up outside my place within the hospital compound. It was one of the two dongas assigned for the island's paramedics and it's where I'd lived for the past eight months. I waited for the dust trail to settle before getting out.

"Thanks again Charlie, I'll catch you later."

"Just make sure you show up on time, Albert'll give you shit if you're late, eh."

I grabbed my gear from the back and gave a wave as I walked away, but Charlie called out, "Oh and Jono, call me when you have a clear head. I've been doin' some detective work and I think I've found your man."

I stopped in my tracks and turned to him. "What man?"

"Mr Wendal, of course."

2

KABUL

Nathaniel Fredericks was staring out the scratched perspex window of the ageing Ariana Afghan Airways 737-400, transfixed by the unfolding spectacle below him. He had drifted into a restless sleep for little more than an hour, before waking with the bright morning sunlight streaming into the cabin. Even though he had secured one of the eight business class seats, the flight attendants were conspicuous in their absence. But at least he had some legroom. After seeing the rows in economy, he doubted he would have fitted there.

Fredericks had spent his adult life squeezing into chairs and ducking door lintels. He was far from lanky, being blessed with a stocky frame that made playing rugby league a natural choice for him. However, a torn cruciate destroyed his dreams of a professional NRL career and he had followed the alternative pathway of a nightclub bouncer, where brawn was equally respected. But Fredericks was more than just muscle. Within a few years he was running the joint, though his current aspirations went well beyond the tawdry limits of the leisure industry.

The plane's inflight entertainment was nothing more than a soiled magazine printed in what he presumed to be Pashto, so watching the ground passing beneath the plane was by far the better option. The arid brown mountains looked like a giant hand had crumpled a piece of paper. Deep ravines and cliffs clawed at the peaks, with the monotonous drab colouration lending a desolate and barren appearance to the landscape. But he couldn't see from an aircraft the real feature that made the country so inhospitable. Decades of civil war, concomitant with centuries of foreign interference and colonial exploitation had wrought havoc with the Afghan psyche. The mismatch of peoples that lived in this patchwork nation were used to eking out an existence. They were only too familiar with the cruelty, death and destruction that prolonged armed conflict leaves in its wake. No wonder some were prepared to risk everything and part with their family's life savings to escape.

There was a 'bong' and the fasten seatbelt sign lit up, followed by a crackling announcement that they were starting the final descent. He raised his seat and gave a comforting tug to the already secured buckle. The plane had cutting-edge technology back in the eighties, but now it looked archaic for 2013. This promised to be an interesting landing.

The mountains outside the window gave way to a parched floodplain with a mosaic of dry-stone walls that grew in frequency and intensity. More complex structures appeared among sealed roads and the country passed from the Middle Ages into at least the twentieth century within the blink of an eye.

The landing gear locked into place with a loud thud and the aircraft began to shake, judder and creak as the wing flaps extended to slow the plane's airspeed. Fredericks glanced across the aisle at the swarthy man in a grey business suit, who was now bent forward in his chair, his eyes tight shut. He had a trimmed black beard that was greying around the tip of his chin, which oscillated in response to his silent incantations.

Fredericks looked back out the window and rubbed his own greying goatee with his right hand. If he had a religion, he guessed that the current circumstances would cause him to ask for divine intervention. But being a devout atheist he smiled to himself. At least if he was wrong and there was a god, then the other guy's prayers should have him covered.

It was his first trip to Kabul, but he had done his research, knew his market and had established several contacts. Two days were all he had to endure and then he would be out of this hellhole. If he had the choice, he would have preferred to stay in Sydney, but some meetings had to be face-to-face.

Soon airport buildings were rushing by in a blur as the wheels bounced on the tarmac with little grace. The landing caused the fuselage and the passengers to shudder, both with the impact and the relief of returning to terra firma. The engines whined in reverse, slowing their speed until they were taxiing away from the runway and over towards the terminal.

He unclipped his seatbelt, despite instructions to the contrary, and stood to stretch out his right leg. His old injury always gave him grief when he sat for any length of time. In the distance a brown haze shrouded the view of the capital. He guessed it was the Kabul smog. He remembered reading about it, but now had to face the reality of breathing some of the most polluted air on the planet. Not even Beijing's infamous opaque atmosphere could compete and that metropolis had over six times the population of this Afghan city.

Fredericks grabbed his carry-on bag from the overhead locker and limped off the plane, ignoring the false smiles from the flight attendants, who had finally made an appearance. He paused on the top platform of a set of airstairs that had seen better days and looked out over the distant mountains. The view was surreal with only the tips visible, the peaks appearing to float above the smog. He sighed, shook his head and walked down onto the asphalt and into the waiting shuttle bus.

His passage through customs was smooth, the journey being pre-greased with cash supplied by his fix-it man, Jangi. With no checked-in luggage, he was soon exiting the secure area and walking out into the arrivals, the pain in his knee having subsided. The building reflected a distinct Soviet influence, austere architecture favouring functionality over flair. Not wanting any delay, he made a beeline for the exit, but as he approached the glass doors, the sight of a man waving a large hand-written sign in his direction, filled him with despair. Anyone who cared to look could see the name 'Mr Fedriks'.

He groaned to himself and did his best to ignore the man, pushing past him and out into the dusty Kabul air. The man slotted in behind Fredericks and said in a low voice, "Don't turn to me, keep walking. Get in the fifth taxi, I'll contact you at the hotel."

Fredericks took a few more steps, then the anger swelling inside him overcame his caution and he swirled around to berate the man for being so foolish with the sign. To his surprise he had disappeared, so he masked his direction change by reaching into his bag for a pack of cigarettes. After lighting up, he inhaled on the smoke, while he scanned the faces in the crowd through his dark sunglasses. He shrugged to himself; if he had to breathe polluted air, he may as well get something out of it. From what he could determine, using all the reflections available, no one was paying him any attention.

Flicking the butt on the pavement, he walked over to the

taxi rank. None of the drivers seemed to mind when he bypassed the first four and climbed into the back of his assigned car. Like most of the other vehicles, it was a beat up Toyota Corolla at least twenty years old. The bodywork was a mixture of yellow paint, dents and rust, with white-coloured doors.

The interior was also dishevelled and as he sat on the tattered vinyl seat, it released a pungent combination of stale tobacco and body odour. Beside him was a hessian rucksack. Without a word, the driver left the rank and headed away from the terminal. Fredericks reached inside the bag and pulled out a long-sleeved brown robe and a flat circular Afghan cap. He threw them on the seat and then withdrew a black form-fitting Kevlar vest with an integrated underarm holster. Below that was a US military M11 compact semi-automatic, along with two 15-round magazines. He nodded his appreciation. At least Jangi had come up with the goods.

He took off his jacket and stuffed it into his cabin bag, before donning the vest, robe and hat. Then he reached for the pistol and, using the heel of his hand, slotted a magazine into the gun. There was a satisfying click and with a fluid motion, he racked the slide to chamber a round and holstered the weapon. The driver didn't even glance back.

It took over forty minutes to cover the ten kilometre journey to the hotel in what made up downtown Kabul. Fredericks spent his time pondering the dilemma of whether it was better to travel with the windows up or down. Open sewers bordered the congested pot-holed roads and all the vehicles, sometimes six lanes per carriageway, were belching out black smoke, even while idling in the stationary traffic. The onslaught of both stench and fumes stung his eyes and burnt his throat. But the lack of a fan meant the inside of the sealed cab became so stuffy, only made worse by the long robe and constricting vest.

He opted to wind down the windows and breathe the fetid outside air, sitting with his hand to his face in the middle of the back seat, as far away from either opening as possible. He rued his decision to avoid the private security firms, with their armour-plated Land Rovers, dark-tinted glass and blessed cool, filtered, air-conditioned interiors. However, he needed to keep a low profile. As low a profile as a tall white Westerner can have in Afghanistan.

His eyes darted from one side to the other, half expecting to see the barrel of a gun pointing in his direction every time a car pulled alongside. But none did. At least the driver kept to the inside lane, reducing his exposure to only one window, although that meant they were closer to the sewer.

Eventually the taxi stopped outside a dilapidated four-storey building down a narrow side street. For a moment, Fredericks thought he might be the subject of an opportunistic kidnapping, but nothing happened. The driver just sat there, hands on the wheel at ten and two, staring out of the smeared windscreen. He hadn't said a word the whole trip.

For the first time, Fredericks realised that there were no mirrors in the cab. Neither of them could see each other's faces. After it was obvious they were going no further, he broke the silence. "Is this it?"

There was the merest deflection of a nod, but still not a word. Fredericks shook his head, grabbed his bag and released the door, which creaked a complaint as it swung open. "Well, thanks for the chat."

With that, he stepped out onto the sidewalk and, as soon as he slammed the door, the taxi pulled away.

Fredericks watched the car leave in a cloud of dust and muttered, "Ignorant wanker."

He then turned to face his accommodation. There was a small sign above the entrance written in English and Pashto script: The Half Moon Hotel.

He sighed, took off his sunnies and ducked through the door into a dimly lit foyer. Without thinking, he switched his bag to his left hand, allowing his right to be free to use his gun. A thick layer of cigarette smoke reduced the light inside even further. His hotel would be no refuge from the poor outdoor air. Although the ceiling was low, the space was large and a group of men crouched around a table as they played a game that was a cross between checkers and pool. The two contestants had chalk dust on their nicotine-stained fingers and the click of the counters echoed off the walls.

One of the audience glanced his way, but paid him little attention, his eyes darting back to the game. Fredericks walked to the check-in where a man with frameless glasses and a smart embroidered waistcoat sat reading a newspaper. He was in his forties with a neat beard and a karakul hat perched on his head at a jaunty angle.

Before Fredericks spoke, the man placed a set of keys on the scuffed wooden top. "Room two thirty. He's waiting for you."

His eyes never left the newspaper. Fredericks tapped a finger on the counter before scooping up the keys. Was it just Jangi in the room or was this the meeting he had come for? He found it hard to disguise the sarcasm in his voice. "Any chance you can tell me who?"

There was a loud click from the gaming table and a muted cheer from those gathered around it. The man sighed and flicked the pages of the paper before raising his eyes towards his guest. They were as dark as the muzzle of a gun and he gave a weary look over the top of his glasses. "How many people do you know in Kabul?"

They stared at each other while the men in the corner reset their game and two new players sat down opposite one another. The proprietor was the first to tire of the confrontation and flicked his newspaper again, before returning his gaze to the printed script.

Fredericks clenched his teeth, then walked off down the only passage leading away from the foyer. As he came to the lifts, he hesitated then carried on past them and headed for the stairs. After four flights of concrete steps, he exited the stairwell on the second floor and followed the numbers down the narrow corridor until he was standing outside Room 230.

The upper screw that held the brass zero to the door was missing and the digit hung down below the others. It was symptomatic of the whole hotel. At some point the place would have been well presented, even comfortable, but now it was just tired, drab and dingy. And behind this door was the man who had organised his accommodation.

He could feel the frustration bubbling inside him, like a mental geyser forced up by the pressure of jet lag. He expected more for the amount of money he was paying this bastard. Clenching a fist, he was about to hammer on the door when he remembered it was his room and he had the keys. He delved in his pocket and retrieved the set, before opening the lock with as little sound as his big hands could muster. As the door inched open, the room came into view and he unholstered the M11, entering in the wake of the barrel.

The scene that greeted him was not what he was expecting. The room was as dreary as the rest of the hotel, emphasised by the closed drapes and fluorescent lighting, but on a table sat four laptops, each displaying split-screen views around and within the building. Some images he recognised, not least the one of himself standing with his gun extended. The man from the airport was sitting in front of the computers and smiled at his entrance.

"Salaam, Mr Fredericks. Rest assured, there is no need for your gun. You are quite safe here."

Shah Jangi Durani was a nondescript man of average build and height with the tanned skin of a tribesman and the obligatory beard of most Afghan males. He wore a beige waistcoat over a light-coloured baggy top and trousers, while a hat, like the one he had supplied to Fredericks, completed his outfit. He was easily forgettable, which was no doubt the look he was trying to achieve.

Fredericks stood upright and slotted the gun back in its holster. "At least you know how to pronounce my name, if you're unable to spell it."

"Ah, my sign at the airport. Don't be too hard on me, sayb. That was the signal for my man in airport security. Do not worry, all the video footage of your arrival no longer exists."

Fredericks gave a begrudging nod and Jangi stood, proffering his right hand. "An honour to meet you at last, sayb."

He spoke with a strong accent, but his English was impeccable. Fredericks had an inkling he may have misjudged the man and had to stoop to accept his handshake. Although his hand was far smaller, Jangi gave a firm grip and when he withdrew his hand, he placed it on his chest with a slight nod.

"I hope your flights were not too onerous."

Fredericks flopped down onto a threadbare seat that sighed under his weight. "I've had more pleasant experiences."

He looked around the room and was surprised to see a trouser press pushed against a wall. "Tell me, Jangi, couldn't my money afford any better accommodation than this?"

Jangi had returned to his chair and his eyes twinkled at the question. "Believe me, Mr Fredericks, there's no safer place for you to stay in the whole of Kabul. Those fancy hotels that cater for Westerners may promise a high level of security, but their clientele's nationality is enough to make the buildings a target."

He waved a hand at the laptops. "Here I have access to the hotel's infra-red surveillance system; it's why the corridors are so poorly lit. No one can approach this room without me or the management knowing about it."

He let the point sink in. "Do you remember the men playing carrom in the foyer? You wouldn't have got through the door if they weren't expecting you. And they were the ones you can see. There's over thirty security staff positioned around the ground floor alone. You should be honoured, sayb. This is where members of the Taliban stay when they need to visit Kabul."

Frederick's eyes flared and he sat bolt upright in his seat. "The Taliban? And what assurances do I have that they'll ever let me leave this place?"

"Calm yourself, sayb. You have nothing to worry about. Men like you in the export business are always welcome here."

3

CALLS

I watched as the pressure needle jiggled and rose to the desired level before the dark liquid dribbled into my cup. The first two black coffees had failed to revive me, so I was hoping for third time lucky. Although my head was still pounding, my muscles aching and the slightest movement brought on bouts of nausea, I had to admit it was all self-induced. I would feel much better if I gave myself an anti-emetic and a litre of intravenous saline, but seeing as I refused to provide either to my drunken patients, I could hardly allow myself such a soft option. I would just have to suffer the side effects of my chosen amnesiac.

A rich brown crema had formed at the top of the cup and I sipped the liquid like a junky relishing the first hit of the day. I'd jumped at the opportunity to escape the limelight of Brisbane when they offered me the two-year transfer to Mornington Island, Far North Queensland. What I was not prepared to leave behind was the chance of a decent coffee, so my one little luxury was a state-of-the-art espresso machine. That, and of course my boat. There was no way I'd travel this far to be marooned on an island, even if the sea up here was teeming with crocs. My friend, Scotty, had joined me for the two thousand K trip from Brisbane, but since then we hadn't spoken much, although it wasn't for a want of him trying.

My eyes drifted out the window, over to where my sixteen-foot Easyrider was sitting on its trailer, covered by a canvas tarp. I needed to take her out for a spin. Maybe I would in my next rostered days off, but I was finding more and more excuses not to remove her cover. Amber had joked I was already wedded to my boat when I proposed to her. The freedom I used to feel from flying over the waves just brought on a heavy sadness. I couldn't help recall the way the wind whipped through her hair while she cried with glee. Why did wonderful memories like that now evoke such sorrow?

I sighed and took a gulp of coffee that burnt a path down to my stomach. "Time to go to work, Jono."

The first shift back was a crossover day with the island's other paramedic. It was the same for all single-officer stations, a chance to update each other on the past week's call-outs and deal with any logistical issues. But out here on the island, with a population of a little over a thousand, there was never too much to discuss. Mind you, Albert would always insist on having a formal station meeting to start the day.

Although as an Intensive Care Paramedic, I outranked him on a clinical level, he was the Station Officer. Therefore, in all other aspects of my job, he was my boss. And Albert never missed an opportunity to remind me. To say I've had a chequered career with respect to management is an understatement, and I did try to turn over a new leaf when I arrived on Mornington. But eight months with this officious bastard was enough to make anyone go rogue. HR never answered my question about why the last paramedic left.

On a positive note, I only had to spend one day a week

with him as he often went pig hunting on the mainland for his days off. It was interesting how we both chose blood sports as a pastime, him shooting and me fishing, though, like our personalities, our focus was poles apart. Mostly, he left me to my own devices, but unfortunately today was crossover day.

I swung open the screen door to my donga and walked down the short flight of stairs, before wandering over to the adjacent hospital building, still carrying my cup of coffee. The heat of the midday sun bore down on my head like an industrial laser beam, but the wound on my forehead meant I had to dispense with my slouch hat. After a shower and clean up, the gash was looking a lot better, but I had to pull the skin together with steristrips and cover them with a dressing. Although a couple of sutures may have helped, seeking aid would have elicited too many questions. At least the mozzie bites had all but disappeared.

The Mornington Island Ambulance Station was a grand name for a carport and a single room off a corridor within the island's medical facility, but Albert wouldn't have it called anything else. I walked in through the side door, past the two Toyota Troop Carriers we used as ambulances, and turned right into the small office. Albert was already there typing at the computer and swung round as I slumped into the other chair, almost spilling my drink.

"Ah, Mr Byrne. Glad you could make it. I hope your timesheet will reflect the fact that you arrived five minutes late for this meeting."

"G'day to you too, Albert. You know, in my humble clinical opinion, I think you need to use your next days off wisely and try to get laid. Have you ever thought of flying to Cairns instead of going to Mount Isa to shoot pigs? You could try hunting of a different kind; there's lots of young, impressionable backpackers over on the east coast who might like a local military man."

His eyes bulged more than usual and his face flushed, before he recovered his Sergeant Major's composure. "Did you just tell me to go get fucked? Be warned, Byrne, I don't have to put up with your shit. I know your transfer here was convenient for all concerned, but there's only so many insubordination charges they'll accept without intervening. Am I making myself clear?"

Albert was in his mid-fifties, yet still as fit as a butcher's dog, with leathery sun-tanned skin and a pole up his arse, courtesy of twenty-five-years service in the Australian Defence Force. When he retired out, he joined what he thought was the closest civilian organisation to the military. However, the undisciplined and rebellious nature of most paramedics meant he had to cope with the disappointment of his career choice on a daily basis. At least here, he only had to deal with one other ambo and could get a replacement without too much fuss. It was almost certainly why he'd remained on the island for so long. I guess he'd found his niche.

I took a sip of coffee. "Sorry Albert, you must've misunderstood my intention. I was only voicing a clinical observation that you seemed a little... uptight and could benefit from a bit of R and R. You know how we have to look for the warning signs of hyponatraemia up here in the tropics. Are you keeping up with your electrolyte intake?"

He narrowed his eyes for a second. "Don't give me your medical bullshit. I've known you long enough to recognise when you're trying to wind me up. It's when your lips are moving. I'll be writing a report about this, mark my word."

"I don't doubt it, I'm sure HR will soon have to build a new extension to house my personnel file. They could name it in your honour, the Albert Wentworth Memorial Wing. It has a certain ring to it, don't you think? Anyway, can we get on with the meeting?"

Albert gritted his teeth and his face pulled an involuntary grimace, but he refrained from taking the bait. These sorts of verbal stoushes had become a weekly tradition and they were one of my few forms of entertainment. He gave me a quizzical expression. "What happened to your forehead?"

"Cut myself shaving."

He was about to respond, but shook his head in exasperation. He reached over to a sheaf of papers on his desk and squinted at the top sheet, before picking up his reading glasses. "Right, well, last Friday I was called out to Mrs Bannister for her recurring cellulitis..."

His voice droned on regarding each bullet point on his list, and I slotted my mental gears into park. When Albert had first insisted on these meetings, I spent some time trying to convince him I could read his case sheets and he should stick to the pertinent information that affected the running of the station. When he ignored those arguments, I would turn up late, orchestrate fake call-outs, or hide his notes. But all my machinations achieved was a longer meeting. I soon discovered that sitting opposite and letting him prattle on was the quickest way to get through them.

I looked around the office. The small size of the room was emphasised by numerous rows of boxes taking up one wall, each marked with a neat label and containing alphabetised store items for restocking the ambulances. Movement near the ceiling drew my attention. A sandy-coloured gecko was stalking a large lacewing, making slow measured advances with sinuous movements of its flexible body. The oblivious bug sat there cleaning its long antennae. The whole time the gecko's two bulbous reptilian eyes never blinked nor left its target. Then, with a sudden sprint, the remaining gap closed and the lizard's jaws snapped shut on the hapless insect.

I smiled as the life and death struggle played out on the office wall. It struck me as ironic how this little fella from Asia was once thought to be a threat to the native species, but the perceived enemy became a friend. It preferred the unnatural habitat of our well-lit homes, making our lives in the tropics that bit more bearable by reducing the bug count. Perhaps, like Albert, it had found its niche.

Albert's drone continued and my mind wandered further, spurred by the gecko. For a nation made up of migrants, our society's xenophobic views never ceased to amaze me. The slogan 'Ban the boats' had decided last month's election, even though most arriving that way were legal refugees. I'm sure a few hundred years ago the local Aboriginal people would've loved the chance to ban the boats.

"Did I say something funny? What's with the grin? Are you listening to me?"

I blinked and came back to reality. "Of course, Mrs Bannister's cellulitis."

He glared at me. "That was bullet point one on the first sheet."

"Right... Just winding you up, Albert. I'm all ears, please, continue."

He stared for a little longer, then continued with his monologue, glancing up at regular intervals to check that I at least appeared to be paying attention. It was gone 1:00 PM when he finished and I walked back to my donga, trying hard to shrug off the feeling that I'd lost about an hour of my life.

I made myself a light lunch and sat down to eat in front of the TV. It had taken a while for me to adjust to working on Mornington. It was such a departure from the shifts I used to have in one of the busiest stations in Brisbane. When signing up, I thought leaving the city for a while would give me the time I needed to get my head straight.

But up here, all I had was time. Too much time.

I woke to the phone ringing and knocked my plate off my lap as I sat up, scattering crumbs across the floor. "Y'ello?"

"Is that you, Jono?"

"What's left of him. Shit, Scotty?"

"The one and only, boss. You're a hard man to contact. How're you holding out up there in the middle of fucking nowhere?"

"Not too bad. I get to sleep on day shifts, which puts a certain shine on things. How's it going back down there in the big smoke?"

"Same old shit. Rumour is that we'll be losing more allowances, and the micro-management keeps getting worse. They got rid of the Ambulance Liaison Officers and now automatically make us available once we've been at hospital for thirty minutes, whether or not we're ready. I've ended up with six case sheets to write up at the end of a shift 'cos the cockheads keep sending us more jobs."

"Six? Shit mate, that's more than I do in a week. You need to graduate past one-finger typing, either that or get the hell out of Dodge. Mind you, you wouldn't like it here. Most jobs are within two minutes' drive. You'd be hard pushed to get the Troopie over sixty before you'd have to stop."

"You know me, I'd spend my down-time souping up the engine, and do a few laps of the town before going to the address."

"I'm certain the locals would appreciate your efforts. Anyway, for what do I owe the honour of a call?"

"Well... you know... I wanted to make sure you're doing OK. Especially this time of the year..."

"What me? Full of the joys of Spring, as always."

"Full of bullshit, more like. Look, I know you don't often talk about what happened to Amber and all the other shit, but... I wanted to say, if you need someone, I'm only a phone call away."

I sighed. "Thanks, Scotty. I'm working through things my own way, but I'll resurface soon enough."

"Just as long as you're not drowning yourself in alcohol. I'll stop sending you the booze if you can't drink responsibly."

I felt myself rubbing my forehead as I laughed in response. There was a long pause before Scotty broke the awkward silence. "Is she still visiting you, boss?"

I hesitated before answering. Sometimes I regretted how drinking loosened my tongue. "She hasn't left me yet, Scotty, but it's only been a year."

"I know, I know. Just hang in there. You're missed back here in Brissie, even the management are wondering why they're getting such an easy run of things. Everyone keeps asking if I've heard anything. It's like you dropped off the planet. Have you not thought of going on Facebook, let people know you're still alive?"

"What, and post a photo of a kitten, or one of my latest meal? Nah, I've never understood Facebook; if I need to get in touch with someone I can call, or email them. Seems to me to be full of people wanting to show everyone how wonderful their life is. After that video of me and Boardie went viral, I'm far more fond of anonymity."

"Plus the fact you're a bit of an oldie now, I guess social media's more for us youngsters, hey Grandad."

"Get stuffed, sonny, or I'll beat you with my walking stick. I may be ten years older than you, but at least I've still got a full head of hair."

"Fair call. Anyway, I've gotta go. I wanted to let you know we're all thinking of you and I'm here if you need to talk."

"No worries, mate, and thanks Scotty. It's reassuring to know you're there. I promise I'll get through this, just give me some more time."

"Will do, boss. Best you get back to sleep, I know how you old folk need your naps."

"Go polish your forehead, Scotty. Catch ya later."

I hung up and sat on the edge of the sofa with a smile. It was good to hear from him. Perhaps I was being selfish hiding myself away up here. I wasn't the only one affected by the actions of Boardie. The thought of his name galvanised me into action. I stood and walked to the bathroom, rinsing my face, before looking in the mirror. I was still only thirty-eight, but even I could see how the last year had aged me. Heavy frown lines emerged from beneath the dressing and spread across my forehead, while the crow's feet were now a permanent fixture. My muddy blue eyes had lost their fire, and the whites were bloodshot. That fucker had a lot to answer for.

I sighed, dried my face, and walked into the bedroom I'd set up as an office. Sitting in the swivel chair, I turned to look at the corkboard that covered the main wall. There were photographs and printouts of news reports, along with spreadsheets and handwritten notes. String tied to pins connected related findings, like a web created by an intoxicated spider, and gloating in the centre was a large photograph of the twisted psycho who had screwed up my life. Darren Boardman, aka Boardie, my former Station Officer. The man who murdered Amber and was thought to have killed at least five others, but was no doubt responsible for many more.

I stared at his face for a while, then dragged my gaze away

and searched the wall, trying to spark an idea, a memory, a clue to help track him down.

Nothing.

I'd been conducting the same ritual for months, but so far the only things I'd found were dead ends. The photo pinned up of the policeman in charge of the case, Detective Giallo, made me turn to my computer and check for emails. But there was only junk, so I typed a quick message and hit send. It had been at least a week since I'd heard from him. I turned back to the wall and the first thing my eyes rested on was a news report of the car crash that killed Boardie's family. I must have read it over a hundred times before, but on this occasion the mention of his twin brother struck a chord.

My phone ringing caused me to jump, it was Detective Giallo. "G'day Jono, you caught me at my desk. What can I do for you?"

"Hi Gee, just wondering if you had any news?"

"I only wish I had, mate, but unfortunately not. You know they've wound down the task force. There's only me left working the case, but if I come up with anything, you've got to believe me, you'll be the first person I call."

"Yer, I know, I'm back staring at my wall, looking for leads."

He sighed. "Look, Jono, it must be tough for you at this time, but I'll not let this go. There's always one case that gets under a detective's skin and this is mine. It's like a persistent itch that won't go away. Don't you worry, I'll find the bastard. There has to be some angle we haven't thought of, some mistake he made. No one's that good they leave no trace."

"I was having a thought when you called, it may be nothing."

"Go on."

"Well, you know how he mentioned my brother dying of cancer."

"Yes."

"I don't remember telling anyone about that in Brisbane. A few people may have known I lost him, but not how he died."

"Yes, well, I ran a check on that. It was in your personnel record, which he'd have access to as your line manager."

"That's my point. How was it in my file? As far as I'm aware, they don't do background checks on employees to include dead relatives. Boardie must have added that information himself."

There was a pause on the line. "OK. Why?"

"Just thinking aloud here. From what we know, he used my... issues with management as a reason to set me up as his scapegoat. I'm guessing where it would strengthen his story he added info into my file, in case he slipped up. Then he could always claim he knew something because of his legitimate access to my personal records."

Another pause. "So?"

"My brother died in a small private care home in Townsville. At some point Boardie must have been in touch with them and as they're unlikely to give patient information over the phone..."

"He'd have go there and sign in."

"And maybe use one of his aliases?"

"I'm on it, what's the care home called?"

I gave him the name and he hung up, leaving me to sit back in my chair, still holding my phone. Could it be that simple, or was this just another dead end?

The potential of a new lead had my adrenaline pumping, and I couldn't stay in my office for long. The last conversation I'd had with Boardie kept playing on my mind. So many had seen the hidden video used to capture our confrontation, but no one seemed to recognise, or even care, that my actions had almost killed an innocent homeless man. They had hailed me as a hero, but I felt nothing of the sort, and part of the reason for being up here was to atone for my sins. Mr Wendal, that homeless man, was one of the Lardil people and this island was their homeland.

In an effort to spend some of my nervous energy, I decided to hunt down Charlie, to find out what he'd discovered about Mr Wendal. I called his mobile, but it went straight to message bank, so I walked over to the hospital and jumped in a Troopie, driving away before Albert collared me. It was a short trip to the police station where I popped my head inside the foyer and called over to the island's police officer. "Hey Miles, is Charlie about?"

He looked up from his book. "Oh, hi Jono. No, I haven't seen him all day. You not checked out his usual haunts?"

"Thought I'd stop here first as I was passing. He's got his phone switched off again."

He grinned and rolled his eyes. "Bloody typical. Well, I guess if he's not at home, you could check out the youth club. Failing that, he'll be down the jetty."

"Cheers. My money's on the jetty."

"Mine too."

I drove round the block and pulled into the dirt car park of the youth-club building, but he was nowhere to be seen, so I set off for the jetty. It wasn't far; nothing was in Gununa. I drove along the main drag of Lardil Street and then took a left, and after a couple of turns, I was looking across the beautiful turquoise waters of the Appel Channel, over to Denham Island.

Mornington lies off Australia's northern coast in the Gulf of Carpentaria. It's by far the largest of the thirty-one named islands in the Wellesley Islands Group, and the only one with a town. As I neared the jetty, everything looked so peaceful. Gentle waves lapped against the shore and a few figures sat at the end of the wooden structure with their handlines dangling in the water.

Back to my left was the turnoff for the Leịka Murrin Hotel, known as The Pub. Now a tranquil scene, but five years ago it was a very different story. Back then, most of the ambulance work on the island started around 8:00 PM, when The Pub closed and the drunken brawls started. It was as regular as clockwork, and if you hadn't had dinner before closing time, you were unlikely to eat until after midnight. Charlie had told me the horror stories when he'd assisted Albert back in the day. "Night after night, Albert would drive the ambulance into the middle of the brawl, jump out amidst flying fists and bottles, then drag the worst looking one into the back. We'd take them over to the hospital, drop 'em off and go back to get another. It was like a ferry service, eh. I remembers Albert sayin' that he'd seen plenty of active service, but at least in the military he was armed. Those were scary days, eh."

Now, standing by the Troopie with the bright afternoon sun glinting off the nearby waves, it was hard to imagine what it must've been like. It reminded me of a childhood trip to Europe, when we'd visited a battlefield in France. The rolling green hillsides, blossoming flowers and distant birdsong revealed no hint of the violent history recorded there. The random thought was from a happier time in my life, before my brother died, and with that mental connection, I was back to the present with a jolt.

I wandered out along the jetty, my boots clumping on the thick wooden slats, the smell of the sea heavy in the air. As I approached, Charlie gave me a wave. "Hey Jono. How's ya head? Hope you didn't let Albert put that dressing on, eh."

He was wearing his wide-brimmed Akubra and his police liaison officer uniform - a light-blue shirt with navy-blue shorts. His dark skin made his grin seem whiter as he looked up at me, squinting in the sunlight.

"No way, mate. I don't think he'd piss on me if I was on fire."

"Ah c'mon Jono, be fair. I think he'd use any excuse to piss on you."

"Good point. Got a spare line?"

"Course. Here, have this, I'll set me another."

I sat down on the edge of the jetty and let my bare legs hang over the side, while Charlie prepared some bait and threw in a second line. One of the other men looked over from his fishing. "What happened t'ya head, Jono?"

"Ah, y'know, Pete. Woman trouble."

He snorted and nodded. "Huh, can't live with 'em, can't shoot 'em. S'why I go fishin'." He went back to staring at the sea.

When both lines were set, I turned to Charlie. "So why's your mobile off?"

"I'm fishin'."

"Doubt it'll disturb the fish."

"It'll disturb me. You white folk are so hung up on keepin' in touch, eh. Yet, when you're together you spend all the time lookin' at your phones. You need to learn to chill, eh."

I had no comeback, so, to prove him wrong, I played with the line for a while, feeling for any nibbles. A bird flitted between the struts of the jetty, hunting for insects over the water, and alighted on a nearby post to preen its feathers.

Despite my efforts, curiosity got the better of me. “So what’s this about Mr Wendal?”

Charlie grinned. “Knew you couldn’t keep it up for long.”

“Well, I can’t compete with you. I’d be here all fuckin’ day and nothing would be said.”

“True. Us blackfellas know how to wait, eh. Anyways, I’ll stop yankin’ ya chain. Your mate, Mr Wendal. As you know, that’s not his actual name.”

“Yep. Got it ’cos that song was in the charts when he turned up in Brissie.”

“Right. Well, when you said that, it gave me a date to work with. A few years before that song, there was a guy who left here under a cloud.”

“He told me as much.”

I felt a slight tug on my line, but then nothing.

“Took me a while to piece things together, eh. Few folk would talk about it.”

He paused and I waited for him to continue.

“Y’see, one night he got drunk. Very drunk. Anyways, when he was found the next day, he was in bed with his mate’s daughter. She’d been beaten and raped, eh. Worse still, she was only fifteen.”

He jiggled the line and rubbed his nose before carrying on.

“He was still out of it, so his mate and another fella took the law into their own hands. Beat the crap out of him an’ cut his balls off with a kitchen knife.”

“Ooo. Mind you, I’m guessing most fathers would be tempted to do the same.”

“Well, soon as he could walk, he left the island and disappeared. No one knew what happened to him, but justice was seen to be done, so the whole thing was never reported.”

Charlie yanked on his line, but whatever had been nibbling broke free. “Damn. Bet it’s stole me bait.”

He wound back the line onto the plastic reel and his hook came up empty. He shook his head. "Hate it when they get a free meal, eh."

He replaced the bait and threw the line back in. I was hoping he'd return to Mr Wendal, but nothing came. A fly landed on my face and I wafted it away. "You suggested there was more to the story."

"You're right, eh."

He rubbed his chin, then spat into the water. "Problem with a kangaroo court is the evidence is rarely checked. It was a good few years later that the other fella who helped with the ball cutting hung himself. He left a note admitting to the rape."

"Shit. So Mr Wendal was innocent?"

"Yep. His name is Dwayne Gibson. All these years he's been living with the guilt of that night."

"And drowning himself in alcohol to forget, but always reminded by the mutilation. Fuck."

"Yep."

There was a sudden jerk on my line and it pulled through my fingers at such a rate that the nylon cut into my skin. It was so unexpected I almost lost the reel. "Shit. That was fast."

"Let her run, let her run, eh."

"I know, just want to keep all my fingers."

I stood up and let the reel spin round my open intertwined hands and the blood from my finger smeared across the outer surface of the reel.

"Hey Jono, looks like a nasty cut. Want me to call an ambulance?"

"Don't joke, I've been to less in Brisbane."

"I could get Albert to come and piss on it for ya."

"I'll be fine, thanks."

After half the line had spooled out, I gripped the plastic.

Even then, whatever had taken the bait was still sustaining a considerable amount of pull on the reel.

"What the hell is it?"

"Probably a shark, eh. You'll need to let it run more, or that line will snap."

"More? You tied off the end, didn't you?"

"Of course, I did… I think."

I gave him a look and he flashed his teeth back at me. I let out as much of the line as I could while walking to the end of the jetty to make sure none of the posts got in the way. Whatever it was, it was still pulling on the line, which disappeared off into the channel. It was trying to run to deep water. Everyone there was now up on their feet, gathering around to watch the spectacle.

As the pressure had lessened, I started the long process of looping in the line, all the while the saltwater aggravating my cut. A good fifteen minutes later, my arms were aching and my finger was numb.

"I think you've lost it, eh. It's reelin' in easier."

"Nah, there's still something on the end."

Then one bystander called out. "Look! Out there. See the movement? Must be a shark."

I squinted through my sunnies and caught sight of the shape moving back and forth, dark against the turquoise water. But as it turned, the sun painted its side and there was a shimmer of light.

"It's not a shark. I saw a flash of silver."

"You sure?"

Before I could say anything, the fish answered for me by hurling its body out of the water. It crashed back down with an explosion of white foam in an attempt to lose the hook, then tried to run again. Realising what it was, I let it take some of my hard-won line.

"Holy crap! You see that?"

"Sure did. How the hell did you snag a sailfish off the jetty, eh?"

"Guess I'm lucky."

Before the last syllable had left my lips, the work phone started ringing.

"Oh crap, no no no! Not now. Can you take that, Charlie?"

He laughed his deep belly laugh, grabbed the phone off my belt and listened for a few moments. "That's a shame, eh. You've got a chest pain over at Birri Lodge. Code One. Too bad, Jono, looks like you'll have to give me back my handline."

I kept reeling in the line. "Can't Albert do it?"

"He's on admin, probably shufflin' papers from one side of his office to the other, eh. You're it, Jono. C'mon, hand over the reel."

"It's a sailfish, Charlie. It's a fuckin' sailfish. If the job's up at Birri the patient'll be an angler. He'll understand."

Charlie stood there grinning with his hand outstretched and I hesitated, overcoming the urge to throw the reel off the jetty. I closed my eyes and shook my head, before passing him the line.

"Shit. Make sure you land that fish for me, I want proof this happened."

Pete called out, "Don't worry, Jono. We all saw it jump. We'll vouch for ya."

"Thanks, but that's not much of a consolation."

I stood there, tied to the spot. Reluctant to leave, but knowing I had to go. Charlie kept looping over the line in a smooth rhythmic action, one turn at a time. "Boy, this monster's still lively, eh. You'd think it would be tired by now. It could be a long fight, but there's enough of us here. Trust me, Jono, we'll get your trophy fish. Now go do your job and save a life."

"Yer, yer, yer, I know. Time to pluck another soul from the jaws of death."

I sighed and turned away. As I clomped down the jetty towards the Troopie, there was a thud and a wail from behind me. I whirled around to see Charlie lying on his back with the reel in his hand and everyone looking at me. The line had snapped.

It took me half an hour to travel twenty-five kilometres along the unsealed road to Birri Lodge. Unlike the city, out here any emergency calls away from the town always meant long delays. At first, bashing the Troopie through the potholes and sliding through the dirt distracted me from the frustration of losing the sailfish. A goddamn sailfish, of all things! But then I began to enjoy the drive, and the exhilaration mellowed my mood. I may not have landed the fish, but it made for one hell of a story. Plus, I could pay out on Charlie for months.

The Troopie left a plume of red dust like a four-wheeled comet, so I slowed down as I drove the last stretch parallel to the little airstrip associated with the lodge. The dust had eased behind me as I turned off into the small complex of about ten low-set buildings, nestled among the casuarinas. A man in a fishing hat waved at me and pointed to a covered area, so I parked next to it.

There was a group of people standing around a picnic table where a man sat clutching his chest. I stepped out of the cab. "G'day. Just give me a second while I get my stuff."

I went to the back of the vehicle, grabbed the response bag and defib then walked to the group. As I approached, an elderly man stepped in my way. "Hello my name's Christopher Beetly. I'm a doctor. I think he's having an MI, you know, a heart attack, so you need to transport him to hospital right away. We would have flown him there, but he's our pilot."

Having a doctor on scene can be a blessing, but more often than not, it's a paramedic's nightmare. Their qualification trumps ours, but very few have any idea how things work in the prehospital field. Those that do let us get on with our job.

I wore my most beguiling smile. "G'day Doc, glad you're here. What did his ECG look like?"

"Well, I haven't got access to one of those, do I, but I gave him some of my own GTN spray."

"Oh, right? So what was his blood pressure before you administered nitrates?"

He hesitated. "I don't know, he had a radial pulse, but he needs to go to hospital."

"Not doubting that, Doc, but seeing as I've got all this kit with me, how's about I get a set of obs and an ECG to be on the safe side."

"Well, if you insist, but I think you're wasting time."

I somehow controlled my mounting anger and kept smiling. If he'd wanted a taxi, he could've used the lodge's car himself, but I let it slide. He moved out of my way and I knelt in front of the man holding his chest. "Hi, I'm Jon. I'm guessing you're the patient, what's your name?"

"Lee."

"Right, Lee. What's happened?"

He was a thin man in his fifties with a face that looked like he could only manage a serious expression. "I was sitting here having a drink, and I got this sudden sharp pain in the middle of my chest, going round to my back. Never felt anything like it."

I applied the monitoring to him as I asked questions. "So, do you have any medical problems?"

"Not that I'm aware of."

"Does anything make the pain worse or better?"

"It's agony when I cough."

"You had a cold recently?"

"Yes, was pretty crook for a week or so. On the mend now though. Well, I was until this happened."

"Is the pain worse if you take a deep breath?"

"Yes."

"What happens if I press here?"

I reached over and the instant I touched the margin between his ribs and sternum he flinched. "Ah Christ, that's it."

"Right, sit still while I run this ECG. Relax as much as you can, breathe normally and don't talk just for a minute or two. By the way, how old are you?"

"Fifty-six."

I smiled at him. "Don't talk."

"Sorry."

"Shhh."

The machine churned out its findings, and I passed the strip of paper to the doctor. "What do you reckon, Doc?"

One glance at the ECG had confirmed my suspicions that there was nothing wrong with his heart. He took the sheet and while he studied the lines, I leant over to Lee and whispered, "Stop worrying, it's not your heart."

He leant towards me and whispered back, "Didn't think it was."

"Any cause for concern, Doc?"

"Well, I'll admit it's been a while since I used an electrocardiogram."

"Oh, right. If you don't mind me asking, what area of medicine is your speciality?"

"Gynaecology, but I can't see how that's relevant. Are you going to transport him or not?"

There was a pause where nobody said a thing, but I'm sure everyone thought the doctor's chosen specialty was relevant. I broke the silence. "Right. Well, we'll be on our way as soon as I've given Lee some pain relief for what would appear to be costochondritis."

I looked back at Lee. "Inflammation of the joints between the sternum and ribs. It can sometimes happen after a cold. Painful, but usually dealt with by a course of anti-inflammatories. So… how many sprays of GTN did you give him, Doc?"

"What? Oh, I don't know, about four."

"Right. That'll be why his blood pressure's so low. OK, Lee, you allergic to fentanyl?"

As I gained intravenous access and administered pain relief, I chatted with the other anglers. "I guess you're all up here for the fish."

One large man at the back laughed. "Of course. Not a lot else to do here, but it's been bloody bonza. Never caught so much in my life."

He pointed to the dressing on my forehead. "What happened to your head?"

"Love bite from a shark. Hey, you won't believe what I had on a handline when this call came in."

I then gave them a detailed account of my sailfish encounter and there was a combined howl of dismay when I got to where the line snapped.

"Should've stuck with it, mate. Lee would've understood."

"Well, he might not have done if it was a heart attack. Anyway, how's that pain going?"

"Almost gone. Shit, that's good stuff. Do I have to go to hospital?"

"Yes. There's a few more tests they'll want to do and what I've given you won't last forever. Now, stop your whinging and get in the passenger seat."

I threw everything back in the Troopie and climbed in the driver's side, saying my farewells. But before I left, I leant out the window and called out to the doctor. He tried to maintain his self-assured strut, but as he walked over his body language showed all the reluctance of a Christian asked to go pat one of the lions.

"Yes?"

"A quiet word between two clinicians. Do you realise what could happen if he was having an inferior MI and you gave him that dose of GTN?"

"Nothing much, I expect."

"Well, for future reference, you might've killed him."

I slammed on the accelerator and left him standing in a cloud of dust.

After a bumpy but slower ride into Gununa, I dropped Lee off at the hospital and parked the Troopie in the ambulance bay. I started walking to my donga, thinking of dinner when my mobile rang. To my surprise, it was another call from Detective Giallo. "Gee. What's up?"

"Got some good news and bad news. Your lead, I found something."

"You're shitting me. How did you chase it down so quick?"

"Hey, I'm a cop. I have my ways. Actually, an old academy mate of mine works up in Townsville, so I called in a few favours and he took a drive out to the nursing home. What's more, we were in luck. They keep extensive records and their archives were scanned into a database. When they checked the data, only a specialist and his GP reviewed your brother's file when he was still alive. But about three years ago, a Dr Curt

McAulay accessed them to research chemotherapy treatment regimes. But guess what?"

"There's no record of a Dr McAulay registered with Q Health."

"Got it in one. But there's more."

I could feel my heart racing. "Go on."

"I searched for the name through our databases and drew blanks on criminal records and car registrations. But then bingo! It was used to register a forty-six-foot yacht that was last moored at Scarborough Marina. Have a guess what the name was."

"Not a clue."

"Ready for this? Plan Sea, spelt S-E-A."

"Holy shit! That's what he said. You've forced me to implement Plan C."

"Yep. He's a twisted son of a bitch. Unfortunately, that's where the good news ends. The yacht vacated the mooring on New Year's Day and 'Plan Sea' was ocean-going, so he could've gone anywhere. I'll enlist the help of Interpol to see if the vessel turned up in any foreign ports, but, hey, it's a lead.

"It's the best news I've had in a long while. Thanks Gee. And I appreciate you keeping me in the loop."

"Hey, it's the least I can do. Don't forget, you came to me last year before all the shit hit the fan. I keep thinking if I'd listened to you, perhaps things may have worked out different and a few more people would be alive today."

"Shit, Gee, don't you beat yourself up, that's my preoccupation. I think we both need to face reality, there's only one fucker to blame and you're now on his trail."

"Thanks. I'll be in touch."

The line went dead and I was left staring at the phone.

4

THE TRAVEL AGENT

Jangi had to make a few last-minute preparations before the meeting with The Travel Agent, so he placed a burner phone on the desk and left the room with an apology and a bow. Fredericks then watched the CCTV views as his Afghan contact made his way along the corridors. After exiting the foyer, Jangi walked off down the dusty road and soon melted into the Kabul street scene.

With all the surveillance images now appearing rather mundane, Fredericks stood and paced around the room. He was not happy about being housed in a Taliban stronghold, but if the Americans couldn't find their adversaries, he had to concede the place provided a good chance of remaining undetected. But that presumed he lived long enough to use his return ticket.

All the pacing failed to ease his nerves. The laptop screen mirrored his movement, causing him to check the monitors, so he gave up and lay down. As with most hotel beds, it was far too short for his frame, but at least there wasn't a footboard. He let his feet dangle off the end and crossed his arms over his chest. The bulge under his armpit and the constrictive Kevlar vest provided some reassurance in their discomfort.

He always knew there were risks associated with this venture, but so far they had been financial or judicial. All had been theoretical until he enacted the plan. He had ameliorated most with layers of deception, subterfuge, and shell corporations, distancing himself from the actual operation. Nothing had been physical. Until now. Now, lying on a lumpy mattress in a Kabul hotel room, the risks were so... tangible.

The longer he waited, the more his body yearned for sleep. He had been awake for most of the last forty-eight hours, but his mind was still wired. His eyes darted from one grey image to the next, not sure what he was expecting to see, but mesmerised by the need to check each view. This was the culmination of all his efforts over the past two years. It was the unfortunate, though necessary, point of contact with the dark underworld that would provide the fodder for what he hoped to be a lucrative enterprise.

The recent changes in Australia's political landscape had forced him to change his plans, but the prevailing policies now meant he could demand far higher premiums, which could only improve his profit margin. His eyes ticked from one view to the next, passing time like the hypnotic second hand of a clock.

The rattling sound of the phone vibrating on the desk woke him with a start. His mind had a confusing wheel-spin moment, but then gained traction and he launched himself off the bed, snatching up the mobile and pressing 'accept'.

He recognised Jangi's voice on the line. "Nice to see you could get some sleep, sayb. It's good that you're refreshed, your ride is waiting outside. The meeting is on."

Fredericks grunted a response and hung up the phone, dropping it in his pocket. He felt anything but refreshed. Glancing at the monitors, he could see a taxi parked opposite the entrance with smoke seeping from the exhaust. The corridors and stairwells appeared clear, and the men were still playing their game in the foyer.

Before he left the room, he ducked into the small utilitarian en suite and splashed water on his face. As he withdrew the hand towel, he studied his own reflection. Although his brown eyes retained their lustre, there were far too many wrinkles around them for his liking. What's more, the greying facial hair and salt-and-pepper coiffure seemed to underline his advancing years.

"Well," he said to himself, "If I can pull this off, I can pay for a whole new look." Then, with a grin, he recited his old pre-match saying. "It's time to dance, big fella."

Throwing the towel into the sink, he gave the monitors a last check and left the room with a quickening pulse. Outside the dim interior, the sudden exposure to sunlight caused him to squint, and he had to retrieve his sunnies. The brightness of the day made him glance at his watch as he climbed into the cab. To his surprise it was 2:30 PM. He must have slept for hours.

The taxi pulled away as soon as he closed the door and he realised that it was the same car and driver from the earlier journey. Jangi probably had him on a retainer, or perhaps he was a relative. This time he didn't bother talking, just opened the windows and sat in the middle of the back seat. He had no idea where he was going, nor how long it would take.

An hour later, the cab stopped in front of a concrete housing block with a row of shops at ground level. Fredericks was certain they had been circling the city. They'd cut down alleyways and weaved in and out of the traffic, he guessed to expose any surveillance. Or it could have been to avoid all the security checkpoints dotted along the roads. He was sure Jangi was somewhere nearby shadowing the taxi, but despite his surreptitious efforts, Fredericks couldn't spot any sign of him.

He stepped out of the cab, but this time when the door slammed, the driver remained in place. Fredericks nodded his appreciation. At least that gave him the option of a quick getaway. As he turned, he was confronted by the sight of two women walking towards him on the sidewalk, covered head to toe in light-blue burkas. They bowed and quickened their pace to pass him, and he forced himself to avert his gaze. As he looked away, the spectacle of a nearby meat vendor drew his eyes. It was a small open shopfront, surrounded by a bright-green metal framework. Along the upper span was a row of large rusty-looking hooks, several of which supported the butchered carcasses of some unfortunate animals. He was guessing they had once been goats or sheep, but wasn't sure. The smell of diesel fumes laced the air and a cloud of flies swirled around like the dust and smoke following the cars. Throughout the long taxi journey, his hunger had been building, but like the women in the burkas, his appetite just disappeared.

Before him, juxtaposed between various third-world stores, was a modern glass-fronted travel agency. Airline logos were scattered over the facade, with the vast majority of the writing in English. There was even a large 'Welcome' sign printed in bold white letters on the door. Fredericks guessed the store catered for wealthy urbanites. He presumed that most of the locals here were too concerned about day-to-day living to have the luxury of planning holidays or contemplating overseas travel.

He opened the door and a clean, crisp, air-conditioned atmosphere greeted him. Despite his short time in the city, he had already grown accustomed to the outside smog, and it was a relief to feel a lungful of fresh air. The inside of the shop was like any other regular travel agents. Rows of glossy magazines adorned one wall, while a coloured map of the world decorated another. A man and a woman sat behind a long formica desk that supported three computer screens. They looked up at his arrival.

The man smiled at him and stood to shake his hand. "Welcome, welcome. Mr Fredericks I presume. It's a pleasure to meet you at last. I am Ghulam Hazrat, but you'll know me as The Travel Agent."

He was in his mid-forties with a groomed bush of jet-black hair and long sideburns, but other than that, he was clean-shaven. His skin was a smooth light tan and his perfect gleaming teeth glinted as he smiled.

They shook hands, and the man made a slight bow before touching his chest, mimicking Jangi's earlier gesture. Fredericks muttered some pleasantries then went to sit down in a nearby chair, but The Travel Agent waved him to stop. "Please, not here, sayb. I think it is more appropriate that we conduct our meeting downstairs. Come, follow me and please, leave your sidearm with my associate."

Fredericks stopped in his tracks, though he realised there was nothing he could do. If he wanted to talk, he would have to comply. The Travel Agent read his hesitation. "Mr Fredericks, this is simply a discussion between two businessmen. I fear you've been led to believe the streets of Kabul are far more dangerous than they actually are. But I cannot afford to invite you into my inner sanctum while you are carrying a weapon."

He sighed and nodded his understanding, then reached in his robe and took out the M11, placing it on the desk in front of the woman. She glanced up at him, then looked away, picking up his gun and depositing it in a drawer. In that instant, her looks captivated him. She was wearing a flowing black shirt over black trousers and a simple light-brown hijab that framed her face and somehow accentuated her beauty. But the feature that caught his attention was her eyes; heavy dark borders encircled striking green irises that made them simply stunning. She reminded him of the famous National Geographic cover 'Afghan Girl', though this woman was in her late twenties rather than early teens.

The Travel Agent ushered him through a door in the back wall of the shop, which led to a concrete staircase, and chatted as they descended. "I must say I'm impressed with your disguise, Mr Fredericks. That cloke is known as a chapan and the hat a pakol. You almost look like a local. However, if I may be so bold, you seem to have neglected one minor detail."

"What? I'm white?"

"No, no, sayb. There are many ethnicities within Afghanistan, some of which have fair skin. The point I was going to make was your shoes."

"My shoes?"

"Yes, sayb. They're not covered in shit."

He laughed at his own joke as he opened the heavy wooden door to his personal office. As Fredericks walked in, his clean shoes sank into the thick pile of a sumptuous Persian rug. Centre stage within the small but decadent workspace was a huge carved mahogany desk. An ornate lamp, keyboard, and computer screen were the only items that marred its beautiful polished surface. Tapestries and framed artwork draped the walls, and behind the desk was a large matching bookcase, packed with regimented rows of leather-bound books.

The Travel Agent sat down in his high-backed swivel chair and gestured for Fredericks to take a seat. "Please, sit, sit. My associate, Zarghoona, will bring us some tea in a moment. I do hope you're enjoying your first visit to my country. You should not believe all that the Western media says about us."

"Unfortunately, I'm only here for a couple of days, so I won't have much time to experience your culture. Maybe on my next trip."

"How unfortunate. I would have offered to take you to see some of the sights. But whatever you do, you must visit the Gardens of Babur and the Museum, if nothing else."

"Thank you for the advice, I'll try to fit that in tomorrow. Now, should we get down to discussing my proposal?"

The arrival of the green-eyed woman interrupted their conversation. She was carrying a silver tea set on a matching platter.

"First, Mr Fredericks, you must have some tea. It is an Afghan tradition."

Once she had poured the hot sweet liquid into the cups, the woman retreated, but rather than leaving, she closed the door with the slightest click and stood in front, motionless, her hands behind her back.

"Please, drink, and then we can get down to business."

Fredericks picked up his cup and took a sip as he glanced at the statuesque guard. "I thought, as we're going to talk about... ah... sensitive matters, that our meeting would be private."

"My dear Mr Fredericks, there is nothing to worry about. Zarghoona here is privy to all my dealings. She is, one could say, my bodyguard. In your language, her name translates as 'green'. An apt description considering her eyes, which you have no doubt noticed. But I often refer to her by her nick-name, Tshaarre. It means 'knife'."

He flashed a smile in her direction. "I'm not attempting to intimidate you, sayb, but she has a particular talent for blades.

That Kevlar vest you're wearing fails to cover both your neck and groin and it's no match for her accuracy."

He smiled, placing his elbows on the polished wood in front of him and tenting his fingers under his chin. "So, let's discuss this proposal of yours."

Fredericks shifted his weight within the confines of his chair, and his hand gave an involuntary pull at the collar of his bulletproof jacket. He thought he had concealed his gun and vest, but this man had recognised and neutralised both before their meeting had even begun. He felt like a mouse being toyed with inside the lion's den, and now he was given his chance to squeak.

"Well, as I'm sure you know, I'm an Australian and my country has a tradition for plain speaking. So, I'll be blunt with you. I understand your speciality is arranging travel services for anyone wishing to start afresh in a new country. Namely, asylum seekers and refugees who do not have the time, opportunity, or inclination to wade through the bureaucracy necessary for legal migration. In a nutshell, you arrange for people to be smuggled across borders."

The Travel Agent's face was impassive. There were no signs of acknowledgement nor irritation, but also no denial, so Fredericks continued. "I would like to offer you a new, premium service with a guaranteed delivery to mainland Australia."

The Travel Agent raised both his heavy black eyebrows. "The mainland? Well, that's only possible through forged documents and commercial flights, and I think that service already exists. Unless you have something new..."

"No international flights into Australia, no need to pass through Australian border controls, no need to claim asylum on arrival, no offshore processing. Just a neat delivery to the city of their choice. And all you have to do is find the clients and get them to Bangkok. I will organise the rest."

The Afghan man picked at an invisible piece of lint on his sleeve before replying. “Well, if they don’t fly in, the only other way is by sea and ever since your government started their new border protection policy, the bottom has fallen out of that market. I’ve been forced to offer discounts for bulk bookings. How do you propose to avoid being captured by the Australian Navy?”

“I’m sure you’ll understand that I need to keep the details of my methods a secret. It is, after all, the basis of my business model. However, I can accommodate twenty passengers per trip and I intend to run at least one delivery per month. Do you think you could come up with those sorts of numbers?”

He stroked his chin and flashed another smile. “Well, Mr Fredericks, that all depends on what sort of price you want for this service.”

“Yes, well, I’d like to make it clear that this will be a premium service, which is reflected in the high tariff of twenty-five thousand dollars per passenger.”

“Twenty-five! Ha, my dear Mr Fredericks, that’s well over double the current rate.”

“But ten thousand dollars only buys you passage on a shitty Indonesian fishing vessel where the best you can hope for is to end up at Christmas Island. Most are now being intercepted and turned back, or set adrift in lifeboats. And what do they get for their money then? If they’re lucky, a promise of a free trip on the next shitty boat?”

He shook his head and paused to emphasise the point. “No, sir, the package I’m offering is a single journey to a choice of five mainland Australian destinations. Also, an independent third party escrow agent will hold their money until the passenger confirms a safe arrival.”

The Travel Agent held his chin with one hand while a

finger tapped his lower lip. "Twenty passengers, you say? And what percentage are you offering me for my services?"

"Well, you'll have the outlay associated with delivering the clients to Bangkok, but I understand you already have systems in place to facilitate that leg. For my part, I've had considerable set-up costs, which I'll need to recoup. Then there's the inevitable ongoing expenditure for what is by far the longest part of the journey. I think you would also agree that I'm taking the greatest element of risk with respect to the authorities."

Fredericks rubbed his goatee as if contemplating the mathematics involved. "I think I'm able to offer you fifteen per cent of the ticket price for each customer."

The Travel Agent gave a broad smile and laughed. "But, sayb, without me you don't have a business. If the funds are held in escrow, then the initial costs will be out of my own pocket. You are proposing an unknown and unproven pathway, which I will not only have to sell to my clients, but spend a great deal of money before it's even viable. As such, the figure I was thinking of was more like double what you offered."

Fredericks reached out and picked up his teacup, taking a sip before returning it to the table. "Although you are the man I want to work with, I have other options within Kabul and over the border in Pakistan. However, I recognise that I have to prove myself to you and I detest haggling. It's so demeaning. As a show of good faith, I will give you your thirty per cent for the first consignment, but after that your share drops to twenty until an annual review, when both parties can renegotiate."

The Travel Agent leant back in his chair and rocked from side to side as he stared at the big Australian. It was a while before he spoke. "And when is your conduit open for business?"

Fredericks smiled at the Afghan. “As soon as you deliver the first twenty customers to Bangkok.”

The Travel Agent’s face broke into a wide beam and he stood, reaching a hand across the polished expanse of his desk. “Well, sayb, I guess we are partners then.”

5

LOST

Warm rays played across my closed lids as the sail swayed back and forth in front of the sun, the cooling wind being both soothing and soporific. Lying out on the deck, I felt calmer than I had done for months. The splash of the waves against the hull and the roll of the yacht enhanced my relaxation.

"Hey Jon, can you rub some more sunscreen on my back?"

"Sure, babe, no worries."

I rolled over and raised myself up on an elbow. She was next to me, face down on the hardwood foredeck with the straps of her bikini top draped by her sides. I squeezed out some lotion on my free hand and started smoothing the liquid into her golden-brown skin.

"Ow! It's cold."

"Don't know how; it's been on deck as long as we have."

"Guess the sun's making me hot."

"You'd be hot on a chilly night in Antarctica."

She laughed. "And you're full of shit."

I massaged her back, rubbing her skin until all the white cream had been absorbed.

"Oh, but you can keep doing that."

I raised my leg over and straddled her body, sitting on her buttocks. I could now use both my hands and I rubbed my thumbs into the small of her back, working either side of her spine.

She moaned her appreciation. "Ooo that's good, keep going."

I kneaded my way up her back, my fingers pressing into her muscles and easing out any knots I found. A gull cried out high above us and I looked up to watch it glide past, but then felt a sharp pain in my finger. I lifted my hand to see blood trickling down from a deep laceration.

My vision went into slow motion as my gaze returned to Amber's back. Jutting up to the right of her spine was the metal point of a blade. In one quick movement, I rolled her over. Blood was oozing out around the hilt of a black-handled knife. Her sightless eyes stared up at the sun. I screamed and turned towards the helm where a figure was holding the wheel. I could only catch glimpses of the man, as the sail wafted to and fro. Then I heard his laughter and Boardie's voice called out, "Plan C, Jono, Plan C."

I woke like a thunderclap and sat bolt upright in bed, covered in sweat. Were the nightmares ever going to end? I collapsed down and gazed at the ceiling, exhausted but reluctant to go back to sleep. The early morning light was forcing its way through the curtains, and the sound of a seagull joining the dawn chorus made me shake my head. My finger was still throbbing from the cut caused by the fishing line. That and the news Boardie had escaped on a yacht had given my subconscious plenty to work with. Perhaps sleeping pills were the answer.

I sighed and got up, throwing on a pair of shorts, T-shirt,

and joggers. A dawn run out to Gee Wee Point might put a fresh perspective on the day.

Exercise followed by a cold shower helped wake me up, but I was still waiting for a new perspective to come my way. I was on to my second cup of coffee, sitting in front of the TV news, when there was a rap on my screen door. Frowning, I looked at my battered old diver's watch: 8:30 AM.

I opened the door to find Albert standing on the steps with a stern expression. "Morning' Albert, c'mon in. Thought you were off hunting in Isa."

"I've had to postpone my flight so I can deal with an issue that's arisen."

"Oh."

I waved my cup at him. "D'you want a coffee?"

"No. Thank you."

"Tea?"

"This isn't a social visit, Jon. I'm here to discuss a serious matter of a complaint about your behaviour."

"Really? You delayed your flight for that? I thought you knew I've had more complaints than Microsoft?"

"You need to take this seriously. This is from a doctor who was so incensed by your attitude he felt it necessary to phone his concerns to the Regional Executive Officer last night."

"Phone? Well, tell you what, Albert, you give him a bell and say that if he can't be bothered to put it in writing, my response will be in kind. IE, verbal."

Albert's face flushed red, and he leant towards me with his chest puffed out. "I beg your pardon! You will respond as I see fit. I am the Station Officer."

"C'mon Albert, you're not on the parade ground now. I

know what this is about. I haven't gone to many jobs in the last few weeks and only one had a doctor on scene. For pity's sake, he's a fucking gynaecologist. He may have over forty years experience and is no doubt very good at dealing with women's bits, but it doesn't mean he can go around administering truck loads of nitrates at the first clutch of a chest."

"What are you on about?"

His confusion appeared genuine, and I smiled as I leant back against the kitchen counter and took a sip of coffee. "You haven't read my case notes, have you?"

"Well, I... I was in a rush because of my flight and I... well, I didn't have time."

"C'mon military man. Isn't the number one rule of attack to know your enemy."

He sighed. "You're not my enemy, Jon. You just have a knack for pissing off people in authority. Then everyone has to run into damage control."

I nodded. "True. But there's no damage to control, it's all covered in my paperwork. I may have attracted a lot of complaints, but only one has ever led to a disciplinary and there were, as I'm sure you're aware, extenuating circumstances."

"So, save me the bother of looking it up. What happened?"

"Nothing much, I was called to a chest pain out at Birri Lodge and there was a doctor in the fishing party. He gave about four shots of his own GTN to the guy who turned out to be suffering from costochondritis. Look, I was very polite to him, despite his rudeness, but when I left I may have suggested his treatment could have killed the patient."

"You couldn't let it go, could you?"

"You think I should have? Whatever happened to the Hippocratic Oath? Aren't they bound by the doctrine 'first, do no harm'?"

"But why piss off a doctor? You know full well he won't get investigated. We've both seen the way the medical hierarchy works. As a paramedic, you're never going to win."

I knew he was right, and I touched the dressing on my forehead, which had started to ache. "So what now?"

"I guess, I'll submit a report saying that I've dealt with the matter, and you were shown the error of your ways. Then it's fingers crossed it all blows over."

I gave a shrug. "Here's hoping he doesn't request an apology."

"Why's that?"

I drained my coffee cup and gave him a grin. "Well, he's got about as much chance of pulling a rabbit out of his next patient's vagina as he does of getting an apology out of my arse."

The day was quite busy for an island shift, with a couple of minor injuries I resolved without having to transport anyone. It was around 6:00 PM when the mobile rang for the third time, with a Code One for shortness of breath.

I pulled up on a side road outside a fibro duplex, just past the grocery store, and cut the Troopie's ignition. As I stepped from the cab, the heat of the early evening was still oppressive and I reached back in to restart the engine. At least the vehicle would be air-conditioned when I loaded the patient.

I grabbed the kit and had to push open a little gate with my leg as I walked towards the property. It creaked an objection, and I lugged my stuff to the entrance before calling out, "Ambulance."

A bored-looking girl in her late teens appeared and opened the screen door to let me in. "Evenin' Cheryl, where is he?"

With a tilt of her head, she indicated the back room, then slunk off to the sofa and cuddled up to a youth who appeared a little older than her. Both were transfixed by a game show on the TV, but her boyfriend was holding a large glass of the local illicit home-brew. Despite the draconian laws regarding alcohol, there's often nothing more ingenious than motivated minds and this disgusting concoction was no exception. It was usually made from Weetbix, Vegemite and cordial, all the essential ingredients to start fermentation. Mind you, it may be alcoholic, but it looked and tasted like shit.

"I'll find my own way, shall I?"

They both ignored me, but then I heard a voice from down the hall. "In here."

I lumbered into the back bedroom, bags bumping off the walls, to see a man in his late fifties sitting on the edge of a bed. He was leaning forward, blowing against pursed lips with every breath, the hum of the oxygen pump giving him the soundtrack of an emphysemic patient.

"G'day Michael, you look like you're struggling more than usual."

His black wavy hair was wet with sweat and beads covered his dark-skinned forehead. "Too right... Jono. It's been... a bad... couple o' days."

"I thought I told you to call us earlier."

"Didn't... want... t' bother ya."

"Well, now you're in this mess you know you're gonna get the works, don't you?"

He shrugged his consent. I had attached the monitoring while I was talking and used my stethoscope to listen to his chest. "Jesus, Michael, your sats are less than eighty and your lungs sound like wet gravel. You need to call us before it gets this bad. You been coughing up much phlegm?"

He pointed to the bedside locker where there was a collection of tissues covered in brown gunk. Next to them was a container filled with cigarette butts.

I tapped the ashtray. "You know those things are going to kill you, right?"

"Think.... the damage... is done."

"Mmm, you're not wrong there. Here's a neb of Ventolin and Atrovent; it should perk you up a bit."

I put the strap of the hissing mask over his head and the drugs clouded around his face like the cigarette smoke he'd been inhaling for years. I then prepared the items I needed to gain intravenous access. Although the remote location meant my caseload was less, working on your own brought a fresh perspective to the job. There was no backup, no one to call for help. You just had to get on with things.

By the time I had a line in and gave a steroid shot, his breathing had improved and his blood-oxygen saturation had reached ninety per cent. "Feeling a bit better?"

He nodded. "Much. I can at least talk now. What happened to y'head?"

"Oh, it's Albert's new style of management. I'll just top up your neb and then go get the stretcher. You think you'll be OK for a little while?"

"No worries."

I gave him a pat on the shoulder and walked into the living room where the TV was still on, but the lovebirds were nowhere to be seen. Opening the door wide, I locked the screen in place to allow easy access, then strode out to the ambulance only to stop in my tracks at the rickety gate. The Troopie was gone.

I did a double take, looking back at the house and out to the road, but there was still no sign of my transport. "Shit, shit, shit! Albert'll kill me."

Very few things will cause a paramedic to run. Exceptions

include imminent personal injury, avoiding management, practical jokes, or the end of the breakfast menu at Maccas. But now, faced with this situation, I started to run. Part of what spurred me on was the memory of the last time I lost an ambulance. Although that was due to a colleague leaving my keys in the cab, I copped the blame and the aftermath was made worse by the cops using a stinger to arrest the joyrider. I couldn't afford for my current manager to learn of this latest fuckup.

The ambulance station was just a few hundred metres away and I could jump in the other Troopie, but I needed to make a phone call on the hoof. "Hi Charlie, thank Christ you've got your mobile on."

"Whatcha up to, Jono? All that heavy breathin' sounds like you're with a lady, eh."

"If only. Listen, I think Cheryl and her boyfriend have just pinched my ambulance."

"Shit, Jono, aren't you supposed to lock those things?"

I continued, taking a breath between sentences. "Save the helpful comments for later. It wouldn't be such a big issue if her dad didn't have to go in to hospital. He's pretty crook. I'm going back to station to get the other truck. What I need you to do is find them. The boy's been drinking hooch. I shouldn't have to tell you if they're caught, he'll be in a world of shit."

I paused to catch my breath. "And, of course, if this gets out, Albert will pin my balls to his chest with the rest of his medal collection."

"It's almost worth a call to Isa, I bet we could see the fireworks from here, eh. Any ideas which direction they went?"

"I parked pointing towards the air strip, but they could've gone either way from there. I'd guess left, away from town."

"I'll try there first. Don't worry, Jono, you've got an Aboriginal tracker on the case."

"Thanks, mate. I'll give you a shout as soon as I've dropped off Michael."

I hung up and ran into the hospital compound, grabbed the keys from the office and fired up the second Troopie. I was back out the front of Michael's house within minutes and off-loaded the stretcher.

My patient was still sitting on the side of his bed when I walked in the room, his nebuliser about to run out. "Here, Michael, let me listen to your chest before topping that up."

He turned to look at me. "Took your time. D'ya get lost or summat?"

"Had a problem with the ambulance, all sorted now, though. C'mon, I'll help you onto the stretcher."

Ten minutes later, I wheeled him into the Accident and Emergency entrance of the hospital and one of the nurses came over to greet us. She was a diminutive woman approaching sixty who'd long since given up covering the greys in her bobbed hair. But her eyes retained a youthful sparkle and what she lacked in size she made up for in a fiery spirit.

"Hi Jono. Michael up to his usual tricks again?"

"Evenin' Gloria. Silly old bugger didn't want to trouble us. Again."

She patted his hand and gave it a rub. "When are you going to learn, Michael?"

She then turned back to me, giving my forehead a strange look without asking about the dressing. "How're his numbers?"

"I've got his sats up to ninety on three nebs of Ventolin and one of Atrovent. IV's in and he's had two hundred of hydro-cort. Blood pressure's good and his resp rate's returned to normal."

Handovers were often different when working alongside

small community hospitals, as most of the patients with chronic conditions were well known to the staff. At that point, the doctor joined us. Robert Marsh was in his early fifties, with a receding forehead and a paunch that was winning the fight against diets and fitness regimes. Despite that, he was still a handsome man who was damn good at his job.

"G'day Jono. What happened to your head? Don't tell me, I should've seen the other guy?"

"Something like that, Rob. I've brought Michael in to see you."

"So, you done all the work for me?"

Gloria helped me position the stretcher next to the hospital bed. "I've done all I can, but you've got a few more toys than me. That's why you're paid the big bucks."

"Maybe paid 'em, but my two exes end up with most of my earnings. I thought I could hide from them up here, but they're like a pack of sharks with the scent of money in the water."

I reached over and took the pat slide off its hook. "You won't get much sympathy from me. Don't forget, I've been on your 'little runabout' moored in the channel."

He smiled and winked. "My two darling sharks only get to feast on the leftovers. As I've explained, that little runabout is my legitimate fishing tours venture."

We all worked together to slide Michael onto their bed. "Money sink more like. How many customers have you had this year?"

He grinned. "Just the right number to make it a going concern. Anyway, enough of my woes. How's my latest customer doing?"

"Not too bad at the moment. Probably needs antibiotics, but that's your call."

"Well, Michael, we'll try to keep you off our Darth Vader

mask, if at all possible. I know how you hate it." He leant forward and listened to his chest. "OK, Gloria, can you top up his neb and get a set of bloods?"

While Rob and Gloria busied themselves working on their latest patient, I ducked outside to call Charlie.

"Any news?"

"Stop your worryin', Jono. The tyres of a Troopie aren't that difficult to follow, eh. Looks like they hightailed it out to Dwenty Point."

"Sure you're not following my trail? I went that way to get to that job at Birri Lodge."

"Give me some credit, mate. I can tell fresh tracks when I see them and what's more, I know a bit about this island. If you're young and have a set of wheels, then Dwenty Point's one place I'd be heading, if I was with a woman. Nice view, very secluded, if you know what I mean."

"Well, just try and catch them before they make a mess on my stretcher."

I could hear his booming belly laugh as I hung up the line.

I made myself a cup of tea while enjoying the hospital's aircon, before completing the paperwork in the office. After printing the pages, I returned to the A&E.

"Hey Rob. Here's my report, if you're interested."

"Always fascinated in the prose you string together, Jono. I'll add it to the rest of them in his file, thanks."

"D'you hear what I caught off the jetty with just a handline?"

"I think the entire island has, but it doesn't count if you don't land it. The story's all hearsay and rumours otherwise."

"Yer, yer. At least I didn't have to pay a fortune to have you troll a line off your marlin boat for hours on end."

"Jealousy will eat away at your soul, my friend. Mind you, it's about time I took her out for a spin. Got to have something on the books. You want to come along again? You know I always need someone to bait my hook and top up my drink."

"Need someone to show you how to fish, more like. Wasn't I the one who caught the most on the last two trips? Saved you the embarrassment of returning home empty-handed."

"That sounds like you're up for a little wager. How about a couple of categories, longest fish and greatest weight? Hundred bucks on each?"

"Make it two hundred and you're on. I'm always up for a share of a doctor's wages."

"Right, you're on." He grinned. "I don't like taking money off the great unwashed, but sometimes the riff-raff needs to be put back in their place."

"Them's fightin' words gov'na. Name the date."

"In a week or so's time? It'll have to wait until I get back."

"Why, where you off to?"

"Not just me. Both Jake and I have been asked to attend the World Summit on Rural Generalist Medicine, no less."

"Sounds fancy. Is it somewhere nice?"

"Cairns. You didn't think they'd send us anywhere exotic, did you?"

I laughed. "So, of all the places in the world a conference could've been held, the two Mornington Island doctors go to the closest urban population."

"Yes, but I'm imagining all those bars filled with scantily clad tourists."

"Careful, you don't want to end up with Mrs Marsh the third."

"Hey, my new motto's 'twice bitten, pre-nup written'. No,

the main reason for me going to this shindig is that I'm hoping to influence where the next one'll be held. My vote's for either Tahiti, Rio, or Barbados."

"Oh, for the life of a doctor. Who's covering your patch while you're gone?"

"Dunno. I think a couple of locums are flying in to man the shifts. C'mon Jono, it's only a few days. What could go wrong? We've got an ICP holding the fort."

6

SARDINES

There was a 'bong' from the overhead display and the fasten-seatbelt sign lit up. Ahmad Nasim tightened the buckle round his waist and gripped the arms of his chair. At twenty-five, this was his first flight, and he had found the takeoff to be an ordeal. In fact, this was the first time he had ever left his homeland. As someone who had dedicated his life to studying foreign languages, the irony was not lost on him, but his parents had insisted he leave. To him, it was like running away; deserting his family and friends; abandoning his country. His emotions were in a turmoil, but he knew that to stay would have been suicide.

The plane lurched and his knuckles paled as he chewed on his bottom lip. The flight from Karachi had taken just over four-and-a-half hours, but cooped up inside this metal tube, crammed in with all these people, was becoming oppressive. Although he had grown up with the Kabul smog, he now felt like he was gasping for air. He wanted to stand up and scream, or run for the exit, but knew he needed to keep a low profile.

He closed his eyes and tried to calm himself, but with every new jolt of the descending plane, his panic bubbled up. Then his right ear began hurting, the intense pain distracting him for a while. He started hitting the side of his head in frustration until the woman beside him leant over.

She spoke in slow single words, enunciating each syllable as if she was talking to an idiot. "You need to blow on your nose, or wiggle your jaw with your mouth wide open. Look, see, like this."

She demonstrated what she meant and Nasim thought she looked more of an idiot, but gave it a go. After a few seconds, there was a whining crackle within his head and the pain subsided.

"Wow, thank you. It's cleared. I'm not used to this, it's my first flight."

"Oh, you speak English. Where are you from?"

He realised he had already said too much and his mind thrashed about, trying to come up with a way to end the conversation. "Karachi. I… I have to go to Bangkok to bring back my brother's body. He was executed for sex crimes."

"Oh… I'm… sorry for your loss…"

He cringed, but the woman returned to her magazine and never spoke to him again. He had to clear his ears a couple more times before the wheels touched down. After a short while, he was exiting the Thai Airways plane and enjoying the relief of the wide-open space of the Suvarnabhumi Airport terminal. The elliptical tube-like building, with its glass walls and ceilings, was stunning, and he allowed himself a moment to take in the view. But he was not here to sightsee.

Nasim followed the flow of people and arrived at passport control. Standing at the back of the throng, he looked along the line of customs officials. Where was the one he needed? Red lipstick and a pair of heavy-rimmed glasses. Not one matched the description. He searched again, staring at the faces in each cubicle. Nothing. What was he meant to do now? Panic started to rise again, but some movement to his left drew his eyes and there she was. She had been looking down, cleaning her glasses. Relief flooded his body, and he positioned himself to join her queue. At some point he was sure she would receive her cut of his parents' money.

On exiting the terminal, he discovered the recent rainfall had left the night warm and muggy. Numerous taxi touts hassled him, but they all failed to say the correct phrase, so he kept moving through the throng. Then, as he thought he may have to double back, a man in a grubby hoodie brushed by him and spoke without turning. "Follow me, this is your rite of passage."

He led him to a taxi and opened the back door. Once in, they drove away from the bustle of the airport, but left the highway before the motorway toll road. The traffic was less here, and they turned again before taking a left into an industrial area. As it was night, there were few vehicles and most of the workers had gone home.

After another minute or two, they drove into the car park of a warehouse and pulled up beside a large blue transit van. There were no windows in the back and the glass of the cab was a dark tint. Nasim couldn't see if anyone was in the front.

The driver spoke for the first time since the airport. "Do you understand English?"

He nodded. "Yes, of course."

"Then listen carefully. Enter the van by the side and immediately close the door. Sit in the first available seat and put on this hood. Do not speak. Be warned, it may be several hours before you get out. If you think you'll need a piss, have one before getting in. We will not stop for anything and remember, whatever happens, do not remove your hood. You won't survive to tell anyone what you see. Now go."

He thrust a heavy black cloth bag at him and pointed at the door. Nasim took the hood and nodded his thanks before leaving the taxi, which drove off as soon as he alighted. He turned to look at the van that sat alone, ominous in the brooding silence. The wet bitumen of the parking lot was still gleaming in the streetlights, but the area under the vehicle was a dry, dull grey. He wondered how long it had been parked there.

With some trepidation, he reached for the handle and released the door, slipping inside and slamming it shut. The view he saw of the interior, from the moment before the light snuffed out, became burnt into his memory. Separating off the cab from the back was a wooden bulkhead housing a small video camera, which pointed at the ten seats arranged in rows. At least six were already occupied, with the passengers sitting side by side, each of their heads covered by their own black hoods.

Fumbling in the dark, he found a seat, sat down and, with a slight hesitation, placed the bag over his head. It had a faint smell of oil mixed with tobacco and the cloth irritated his nose, but he would have to get used to it. Sitting there in forced silence, within such proximity, was an unnerving experience. His ears strained to hear the slightest noise from outside, but then the creak of a seat, a sniff, or a muted cough would distract him. The longer he was left with his thoughts, the more difficult it became to shake one disturbing impression. Here they all were, lined up, passive and gullible, waiting for their execution.

It felt like an eternity, but it was about twenty minutes before there was the hum of an engine. Then a pause, a door slammed, and the car drove away. Footsteps. The sound of liquid splashing on the ground. Another pause, then the clunk and grating slide of the door opening and closing, accompanied by the sway of the vehicle.

The newcomer took a couple of steps, then sat down next to Nasim, almost landing in his lap. As a reflex, the man mumbled his apologies in Urdu. As he uttered the words, a command hissed from the cab. "Khamoshi!"

Nasim recognised the Urdu for 'silence'. Evidently there was someone in the front who was not only watching, but also listening to their human cargo. This was going to be a long few weeks, if everything went to plan. He leant his head back and to his relief discovered the seat had a headrest. Fatigue drenched his body, and his shoulders sagged, but try as he might, sleep evaded him. Despite being awake for more than two days, his mind was far too alert.

The road trip from Kabul to Karachi had lasted over twenty hours. Nasim spent most of the bumpy journey lying on a rug in the back of a flatbed truck among assorted produce. He had arrived in Pakistan's largest city feeling battered and bruised, but at least they allowed him to sit in the cab for the rest of the trip.

Now, in the pitch dark with the hood itching his nose, every one of his abused muscles was insistent on relaying its status. Bored, tired, but still anxious, he sat in his seat while the taxi driver ferried two more passengers from the airport to the van. By Nasim's estimate, there were at least ten of them when the engine fired up and they pulled out of the car park.

It took about an hour and a half to reach the huge container port of Laem Chabang on the Gulf of Thailand's northern shores, but Nasim and his fellow refugees were none the wiser. The van had spent the first fifteen minutes circling the industrial estate. After that, they headed off south on Motorway Seven, and onto the Chonburi Pattaya Highway.

Although it was the middle of the night, the port was still a hive of activity, with all the thoroughfares lit by glaring floodlights. Trucks came and went, forklifts buzzed about, while massive cranes loaded containers onto the flotilla of awaiting ships. The blue van was just one more insignificant vehicle in the mayhem of machinery, and no one paid any attention to its passage into a darkened warehouse.

Nasim was still wide awake when they stopped and the motor switched off. As if to rub salt into his wound, the man beside him was now leaning against his shoulder, snoring. Nasim gave him a shove and he woke with a grunt. There were voices outside and the side door slid open with a thud.

"Welcome, welcome dear people, please be patient. You will be led one at a time to your sleeping quarters, but you must make sure your hoods remain in place."

The voice repeated the message in Pashto, Urdu, and Farsi, all of which Nasim understood. Someone off-loaded the first person and there was a wait until the next occupant was guided away. When Nasim's turn came, a hand grabbed him by the arm and, with little ceremony, pulled him out of the van. He was just glad he could stretch his aching legs and start moving again. His guide led him over to some steps, which clanked with each footstep as he climbed the flight, then out onto what felt like a platform. His hands were placed on a set of warm metal handrails. "It's a ladder, climb down. Understand?"

He nodded and descended, passing through a narrow opening, which he discovered by catching his elbow on the heavy edge. It took all his might to suppress an expletive, before continuing through the hole and down to the floor below. Once there, Nasim was told to move against a wall and await further instructions. The guide spoke in faltering Pashto, and the words echoed around the room into which Nasim had climbed.

He shuffled a metre or two in his hood-induced blindness, before he found a wall and turned to rest his back against it. He counted another seven climb down the ladder before there was a low thud followed by a ratchet-like spinning sound. After that, they all stood in silence. Nasim could hear the others breathing, they were that close.

After more delay, a tinny voice announced in four languages that it was now safe to remove their hoods, but to keep hold of them for later. Nasim grabbed at the bag and wrenched it off his head, but then had to blink due to the bright fluorescent lighting. When his eyes became accustomed, nine other faces confronted him, all blinking and looking bewildered. They were crammed together in a long metal room, somewhat like a corridor, about two and a half metres high by just over two wide. A honeycomb of nine bunks took up each end wall. They reminded him of a photograph he once saw of a Japanese hotel. In the middle, set either side into the ceiling, were two more bunks, suspended over a toilet and washbasin.

People already occupied ten of the beds, with only their faces visible, cocooned in their sleeping quarters like bee larvae in a hive, watching them with a mixture of pity and amusement. Nasim had to fight an overwhelming urge to put his hood back on. He could feel beads of sweat forming on his forehead as his chest tightened with every breath. Being in a plane had been bad enough, but this? This was for two weeks! How would he cope?

Without being instructed, he climbed up into one of the top bunks and slotted his body in, burying his face into the pillow. He began conjugating English verbs to occupy his mind. It had been the language he found most difficult to learn, but it was the one he was most proud of mastering. However, it was also the reason he was in this mess.

He was calming when the disembodied voice once more sparked into life, with the first announcement being in English.

"Welcome to our new guests and apologies for the manner of your arrival. It was an unfortunate necessity to protect our anonymity and to hide our delivery method. On that note, may I take this opportunity to remind you that when you arrive at your final destination you should not try to claim asylum, just disappear into your chosen city. If you are ever caught, show them the flight ticket stubs we've provided and tell them you discarded your fake passport. Reveal nothing about your actual mode of entry. Please be warned, we do not appreciate anyone who crosses us and we have contacts in the immigration processing facilities who are prepared to exact any required retribution. Let me be quite clear, if you talk, you will not survive long enough to enjoy any claimed asylum.

"Now, to more pleasant matters. Regarding your accommodation, as you can see, there isn't much floor space for all of you to be out of your beds. So, pick a bunk and try to spend most of your time in it.

"If you are struggling to understand this announcement, we'll repeat it in your native tongue. We've supplied each bunk with an English phrase book, which we would encourage you to use and learn. You'll also find twenty containers of liquid protein mix. Don't worry, it's all halal.

"Please be aware that the journey takes about two weeks, so you need to ration yourselves. The liquid has been formulated to provide your bodies with what you need and also limit your… output. We understand that what you need to survive may not be what you want, but it's just for two weeks.

"The liquid gives you some fluid, but there is a tap next to the toilet with drinking water. Again, ration yourselves.

"Everyone has two pots of different coloured tablets. Take

two of the pink ones each day; they will help with any nausea. If you get anxious, or want to sleep, take two of the white ones.

"Keep any noise to an absolute minimum and do not bang on the walls. The room is insulated, but there is no reason to alert the authorities to your presence. Please be aware, we can watch you and talk to you, but two-way communication is only possible in an emergency. If one occurs, press the red button on the wall near the entrance. You might not get a response, but we will be monitoring the situation.

"Thank you for listening and I hope your journey is not too arduous."

The voice droned on, repeating the instructions three more times, but Nasim was already hunting out the white pills. He took two and washed them down with a mouthful of protein mix. Holding the pot up, he doubted there were enough tablets to last him a week, let alone a fortnight.

Outside the modified shipping container, the man with the mic released the transmit button and began packing away the radio link. "Right, they're all good to go. Let's get this box out to the gantry crane so we can load it on the ship. Next stop for them is Merauke."

A nearby colleague shook his head. "It's a long fuckin' way to West Papua. D'you think they know they'll be drinking their own piss?"

He looked up from his work with a grin. "Hey it's filtered and anyway, I don't give a shit. I'm just glad it's not me in that sardine tin."

7

CRAZY

It was Sunday afternoon, and I'd driven the Troopie down to the water for a bit of fishing. I was sitting on the jetty in my uniform with a handline in, the sun warm on my bare arms and legs, when Charlie came loping down the walkway towards me carrying a bag.

"G'day, Jono. Tryin' to catch another sailfish?"

"Not being that specific. Anythin'll do. Must say, the Troopies have never been so clean. What did you say to the lad?"

He sat down beside me with a grin. "Island justice, my friend, island justice. The young Mister Johnson has to keep both ambulances pristine for two months before he's allowed to spend any time with Cheryl."

I nodded my appreciation. "Brutal, but fair."

"Kept him out of the lock-up and he'll think twice before stealing another ambulance, or any other car for that matter, eh."

"Just make sure he doesn't tell Albert what happened."

"Don't worry, he's sworn to secrecy, mate."

Charlie pulled out a handline and some bait from his bag and was soon fishing next to me. We sat there in a comfortable silence as a group of kids appeared at the shoreline, laughing as they played tiggy.

Charlie spoke without looking up. "You miss the city?"

I thought for a while as I looked out across the turquoise waters, golden sand, and cloudless azure blue sky. "I'd be lying if I said I didn't, but this place grows on you."

"Has that effect on people, eh."

Another ten minutes slipped by before Charlie again broke the silence. "Looks like you'll have a scar on your forehead."

"Glad I could get rid of that dressing. At least I can wear my hat now. What's with you today, anyway? You're being unusually chatty."

Before he could answer, he yanked his line and stood up to reel it in. "Got somethin' decent on the end of this."

"Don't snap the line."

He shot me a look, and I tried to maintain my innocent smile. Within a few minutes he was pulling up a good-sized coral trout, the mouth of the bright-red fish gaping as it left the water. Charlie guided his prize onto the jetty and, before it flopped about, whipped out a wooden rolling pin and hit the fish's head with a crunch.

"Hey, hey. What a beaut. There's Sunday dinner sorted out, eh."

"Guess you don't lose 'em when they're your fish."

"I'm yet to lose an ambulance, eh."

"Touché."

Just then, there was a squeal, followed by a big splash as one kid jumped from the jetty. The others ran from the shore into the sea and the whole group began splashing and laughing in a frenzy of white foam, stirring up the clear waters.

I looked up at Charlie. "I didn't think it was safe to swim here?"

His forehead buckled in a row of furrows as he watched the children. "It's not. They only swim when they've forgotten about the last attack and that was some time ago, eh."

He waved the rolling pin at them as he walked back along the jetty. "Hey, kids. Out the water. C'mon, you've had your fun. It's too dangerous, eh."

They ignored him for a while, but he kept calling down to them, standing on the jetty like a patient lifeguard. One by one they heeded his warning and slunk back up the shore, water dripping from their near-naked bodies. They stood in a group, their arms in front of their chests, elbows together, clenched fists covering their mouths, as he used the rolling pin like a conductor's baton.

"You guys should know better, especially you Zac Bateman. You were swimming here when Bella was taken, eh. That was less than a year ago. Do you have such a short memory? Go on, be off with the lotta ya."

He turned and started walking back towards me with a smirk, patting the rolling pin in his hand, when there was a splash from behind him. Zac had thrown himself backwards into the water and was flailing his arms in mock distress. The other kids laughed and Charlie shook his head before turning to deal with them.

Seeing him coming back, the boy stood up and made to leave the water, but the sea rose around him like a mini tsunami. Before he could scream, he was lifted and thrust forward towards his group of friends, who scattered backwards away from his wide-staring eyes.

As the wave drained away, the immense body of a huge crocodile lay partially exposed on the beach, its jaws clamped around the boy's hips. The surreal scene seemed to stop like a freeze-frame, but water still drained off the reptile's armoured skin as the deafening silence rang in my ears.

Then time caught up like a sonic boom. I leapt to my feet. The boy started screaming. The kids echoed his cries. And the croc began to slide back. But it was Charlie who moved first. He sprinted down the jetty and launched himself full stretch off the structure, with his arm held high. I mouthed "No" as he belly-flopped in the water next to the beast and his wooden rolling pin smashed down hard across its eyes.

The animal opened its jaws wide, throwing its head away from the assault, and dropping the boy's body in the shallows. Charlie sprang to his feet and stood between the predator and its prey. He yelled at the top of his voice and brought his makeshift weapon down for a second blow, this time connecting with the croc's nostrils.

The monster snapped once towards its assailant, then with a swirl of its tail, sank back under the waves. Charlie stood there, knee-deep in blood-stained water, his legs wide and the rolling pin held out in front of him. I'd started running as soon as he leapt off the jetty and I was now sprinting across the sand towards the boy. I scooped him up in my arms, as best I could, and carried him away from the water's edge, calling back to my friend. "Charlie, move you crazy bastard! Go get the stretcher out of the Troopie."

He made one last scan of the water, waving the rolling pin like a corroboree dancer, before moving backwards up the beach, then ran past me to the ambulance. When I caught up, I laid the boy on the stretcher and started cutting away his blood-soaked shorts. Zac kept trying to sit up, his eyes as wide as a barking owl's.

"Lie down, Zac. Try to keep calm. The croc's gone. Don't worry, let me check you over."

His pulse was fast, weak and thready, and he was panting

to breathe. A series of holes ran across his lower abdomen and upper thighs; his right femur looked broken. I grabbed a small pelvic binder from the back of the truck and threaded the wide band under his legs so the device encircled his hips.

"Here, Charlie. Pull on that loop for me."

The buckle clicked, and I locked off the strap. His pelvis was almost certainly fractured and if I didn't stabilise the structure, he could soon bleed out internally from an injury like that. I reached into the kit and pulled out a bag of saline, cutting off a corner with the shears from my belt. The sooner I could clean his injuries, the better.

"Grit your teeth, Zac, this might sting."

I motioned Charlie to hold his upper body, then poured the liquid over the open wounds. The boy began whimpering, but otherwise lay still.

"Right, give me a hand to load him. Here're my keys, I'll work on him in the back while I call the hospital. You drive and call Miles to come deal with these kids."

"On it, Jono."

I turned to the group of terrified children. "Move back up the beach and wait there. Someone'll be here soon to look after you."

"Will he be OK, mista?"

I didn't have time to console them and called out as I jumped in the ambulance. "I'll do everything I can."

Working on a patient in a Troopie is always difficult, but Zac needed to be in hospital. Staying to 'play' on scene was pointless. I somehow attached monitoring and gained intravenous access while calling the A&E, my phone held between ear and shoulder.

"Hi it's Jono, who's that?"

"Gloria."

"Good. I'm bringing in a ten-year-old boy from the jetty. He's been grabbed by a croc."

"Shit."

"Yep. And it was a big one. I think he's sustained at least one femur fracture, likely pelvic involvement, and abdominal injuries. There are several significant puncture wounds back and front. Blood pressure is ninety systolic, heart rate one forty. We'll be with you in a minute or two."

I dropped the phone so I could secure the wide-bore cannula I'd jabbed into a vein, but refrained from attaching a bag of fluid. What he needed now was blood. I kept talking to him as he stared at me.

"You're gonna be fine, Zac, you're doing great. You'll be in hospital in a few seconds. I put that needle in your arm so I can give you something for the pain. You'll be fine."

To be honest, I had no idea what his chances were, but they were a hell of a lot better than before Charlie intervened, so I wasn't worried about lying to him. Yet his reply floored me for a second.

"What 'bout me brutha? I'm not supposed t' leave him."

My mind reeled back to my own brother and how helpless I felt when his cancer was first diagnosed. And here was a kid who'd just escaped the clutches of a croc worrying about his younger sibling.

"Don't worry about him Zac, Charlie's sorting that out and he'll call your parents next, OK?"

He nodded. By the time Charlie reversed into the hospital car park, I'd finished drawing up some fentanyl when Gloria flung open the back door.

"Let's go."

I gave him his first dose of pain relief as we wheeled him into the A&E and made our way to the nearest bed. Other than Gloria, there were already two concerned-looking nurses

I recognised waiting at the bedside, and then a new face came running in from the ward. She was in her late twenties, slim with dark brown hair tied in a long plait and large circular heavy-framed glasses. Her choice of clothes was more suited to a night out on the town than an outback hospital.

She looked straight at me. "I'm Dr Gibson. Are you sure this was a croc attack?"

I glanced at the boy's body with its two parallel rows of huge puncture wounds, then back at her. "Yes. We witnessed it. That crazy bastard behind you saved his life by belting the croc with a rolling pin."

The doctor turned to Charlie, who had followed us in and he gave a sheepish grin. She faltered for a second then turned to me. "Right. What're his obs?"

"Let's get him on your bed and I'll give you a handover."

As soon as he was transferred, the nurses started applying their monitoring. As I spoke, I gave another dose of fentanyl. "This is ten-year-old Zac Bateman. He was grabbed while in knee-deep water by a very large croc that bit him across his hips. He was held in its jaws for less than ten seconds, before being dropped into the water. There was no rolling, no shaking. I manhandled him onto the stretcher where I applied a binder to support his pelvis, which looked unstable. Other injuries are the right femur, which appears fractured, and the obvious puncture wounds, which I've irrigated with a litre of saline. He's got a sixteen gauge in his ACF and he's now had fifty micrograms of fentanyl. I haven't given any fluid because he's maintained a radial pulse and both feet are well perfused, but his BP's around ninety."

I took a breath. "As to other stuff, he doesn't think he's allergic to anything and says he's normally fit and well. Last thing he ate was breakfast at eight, and I think Charlie got a message to his parents on the way here."

I turned to Charlie, and he nodded his agreement. "They're on their way, eh."

The doctor clicked into gear. "Right, let's get some more pain relief administered, bloods drawn, and I'll organise a transfusion, antibiotics, ultrasound, and X-rays. Can someone call for a medevac?"

"I'll give our people a ring. I'm not sure if you're aware, but it'll take at least two hours before the plane arrives."

"Right. Rob warned me about the delay, but thanks."

"After I've called, do you want me to apply a traction splint to that femur?"

"Sure. Yes, please."

We burst into a hive of activity around the boy's supine form. However, despite the clinical focus, the nurses still had time to talk softly to Zac and offer him as much comfort and reassurance as they could while performing their tasks.

Once the splint was in place, I walked over to where the doctor was studying the X-rays. I looked at the grainy black and white images over her shoulder. "Well, the pelvic binder looks like it's in the right position. At least his vertebrae appear intact."

"Yes. I'll get another view of his femur with that traction splint in situ, but I'm more concerned about the rectal and urinary bleeding."

She paused, then turned to me holding out a hand. "You must be Jono. I'm Lydia, pleased to meet you. Rob said I should trust your judgement."

I raised my eyebrows. "High praise indeed. I thought he had me down as another dumb ambo."

"I think we both know that's not the case." She smiled. "Well, I'm no expert on crocodile bites, but from what I understand, infection is a major issue. I've given him the works with respect to antibiotics: ceftriaxone, metronidazole, and doxycycline, and he's also getting a tetanus jab for good measure. He's going to need a urinary catheter, but I'm wondering whether it's worth putting him under first."

She hesitated. "It's just... I haven't done many RSI's outside my theatre placement, and those were with an anaesthetic team."

I rubbed my chin. "The staff here have assisted with them, and I've got plenty of experience of prehospital intubation from Brisbane. If you wait for the flight doctor to arrive, it would mean delaying the medevac. I'm sure it would be better if he was intubated for the flight. It's at least four-and-a-half hours to Townsville from here. If you want, I'll phone a friend and ask her opinion. I've got a direct line to our Head Medical Officer, Dr Sarah O'Driscoll."

I took out my mobile and tilted my head to one side.

She hesitated for a moment, then nodded. I turned and walked away as I dialled the number. After a few rings, a voice answered. "O'Driscoll."

"G'day Sarah, it's Jonothan Byrne here."

"Hello Jon. Heard you're still causing waves up there on Mornington. Just had to deal with your latest complaint."

"The one from the gynaecologist? He was an arse."

"I know. I told him as much. Is this call about the crocodile attack?"

"Jesus, you do have your eyes and ears everywhere."

"I was informed as soon as you requested the medevac. What's the problem?"

I gave her a rundown of the situation and she listened without comment. When I finished, there was a long pause. "Are you still there?"

"Yes. The boy needs an RSI. Make sure you run the show, but don't annoy the doctor. Call me when you're done. Oh, and Jon."

"Yes?"

"Don't miss the tube."

The line went dead and I looked at the mobile. "Nothing like pressure."

Despite the high stakes, we performed the Rapid Sequence Induction with no issues. Once I secured my tube in his trachea, the doctor set up a respirator and the machine began breathing for Zac. With at least three syringe drivers running and a blood warmer delivering another unit of packed red blood cells, the boy's well-being was now firmly in the realm of the hospital staff.

I stepped back from the bed and left to look for Charlie. He was sitting outside on a bench and I sat next to him without a word.

Charlie was the first to speak. "Bet my coral trout's gone by now, eh."

We looked as each other and started laughing.

"You've lost another bloody fish. Believe me, I've seen some crazy things in my time, but your jump was one of the craziest. Who d'you think you are, Crocodile Dundee? At least he had a huge knife when he took on a croc."

He shrugged. "Didn't have time to think."

I did my best Paul Hogan impersonation. "That's not a knife… This is a knife… Oh, no, hold on, it's a rolling pin."

We both laughed again.

"Ah mate, crocs are lazy, eh. They're after an easy meal. Put up a fight and there's a chance they'll let go. How's he doing in there, anyways?"

Although Zac was in a critical condition, I wanted to remain upbeat for Charlie's sake, and the boy's family, along with the rest of the community who'd no doubt contact him. "Well, other than the wounds from the teeth, his pelvis is fractured in two places, he's got a broken leg and his bladder and bowel might be perforated. But thanks to you, he's still alive and in with a good fighting chance."

"Anyone would have done it, eh."

"No. That's just it Charlie, they wouldn't. If you hadn't jumped in waving your rolling pin, he'd have been crocodile shit for sure. You're a fucking hero, mate."

He grinned at me and I slapped him on the back as my mobile rang. "Oh Christ, that'll be the Big 'O'. I've gotta take this call."

I pressed accept as I walked away. "Hi Sarah, sorry for the delay, I had a few other things to deal with. The RSI went like clockwork, an easy grade one view and I got a size six tube in. The doc's happy and packaging up the patient for the flight."

"Good. It's been a few months since your last tube." There was a pause on the line. "You know you're wasting your time and skills up there on Mornington."

"Well, no one was in a hurry to stop me leaving. I think it suited all parties at the time."

"Perhaps. When are you coming back to Brisbane?"

"Depends if you can offer me a position on one of the ICP cars."

"You know I can't promise that. Just do me a favour and don't spend too much time out rural. You'll get rusty."

With that, the line cut and once again I was left staring at my phone.

8

HOOKUP

A green glow from the screens lit Matthew MacNair's face as his eyes focussed on the single radar blip. They were approaching on a collision course. His right hand flexed on the throttle as he maintained the revs just in the red, while his left kept the wheel steady.

"You gonna ease up soon, Matt? You don't want to swamp 'em with our wash."

He darted a look at his brother, Luke, before returning his gaze back to the navigational screens. He spoke in a low grumble, barely audible over the roar of the diesel engine. "Best you get yourself and that useless mate of yours down to the deck, unless you need remindin' who's the fuckin' skipper."

The younger man pushed himself off the chart table and flicked the stub of a joint out a side window. A burst of sparks flared against the black night's sky like a tiny firework as the wind whipped it away. "Aye aye, cap'n."

"And don't forget, you've only got ten minutes to swap the hawsers and re-couple the umbilical. We can't afford for you to fuck this up, Luke."

He paused as if he was going to reply, but changed his mind. The older brother sensed the hesitation and regretted his harshness. "Look, just remember how we've practised it and you'll be fine."

He nodded. "Don't worry, Matt. It'll be..."

"There they are!" His brother interrupted, pointing out the windscreen.

A small light waved in the inky darkness, like a sky lantern lost in the void. Matt eased off on the throttle and spun the wheel, causing the twenty-metre trawler to lurch over to one side. Despite the size of the vessel, he handled her like a racing dinghy. Within seconds both Luke and the other deckie, Bruce, were fending off and throwing lines to a large wooden Indonesian fishing boat that was wallowing in the swell caused by their arrival.

Once secured, the crews of both boats busied themselves with their rehearsed tasks, while Matt watched from the bridge. He considered bathing the scene with the floodlights, but decided not to. It would make the work easier, but the less attention they attracted the better. With that thought, he went back inside and checked the radar. Nothing within at least ten nautical miles. At least on the water's surface. He had to hope there were no Navy drones in the sky. On impulse, he walked outside and looked up, but then snorted a laugh. One of those spy planes could film their rendezvous from an altitude of over fifteen kilometres. It was like looking for a sniper in the pitch dark.

He checked his watch and blew hard on his thumb and index finger, creating a shrill whistle that cut through the clamour on the deck. Luke looked up and Matt spun a finger at him. His brother nodded and ran his checks before giving a thumbs up.

Matt watched as the last Indonesian left and released the

mooring lines. He then engaged the engine and increased the throttle, taking the strain of their submerged cargo and pulling away from the other vessel that was already hurrying from the scene.

Luke joined him on the bridge, grinning. "Seven minutes and twelve seconds, Mattie boy. How could you ever doubt me?"

"Well, you might've bought us some time, but there's now only thirty-four left and this old girl is handling like a bitch. The best I can get out of her is five knots. We gotta hope you connected the fuckin' umbilical right 'cos I need you to fire up the motors on the rig."

Luke looked crestfallen, but did as his brother instructed, lumbering over to a battered old fishfinder and releasing a clip on the side of the unit. The screen swung away to reveal a shiny new collection of lights and switches, along with a large red button protected by a clear plastic cover. At the flip of a few switches, the corresponding lights glowed green, and he replaced the phoney monitor cover. "Fingers crossed, but that should make a difference in a minute or two; you've got to wait for the props to get up to speed."

"You better be right 'cos we're fucked if that VMS pings when we're outside Australian waters."

He pointed up to the ceiling way above which was the transmitter for the Vessel Monitoring System, attached to the mast. It sent a signal to a satellite every hour and was a legal requirement for commercial fishing boats. Although their venture was far from legitimate, trawling was part of their cover, and so the VMS was an ironic essential to prevent undue scrutiny.

As they steamed towards the invisible line designating Australian territorial waters, the tension on the bridge was palpable. Despite the recent refit, the engine whinged like a sunburnt pommie. But ever so slowly, their speed increased and soon they were crashing through the swell at a respectable nine knots.

Matt took his eyes off the array of screens for a second to give his brother a begrudging nod. Luke grinned back, knowing it was the best praise he was likely to get. The two of them remained in silence, bracing and swaying in unison with the sideways roll and undulating roller-coaster pitch of the vessel. After a while, the older brother snatched up the intercom and called the deck. "How're things holding down there, Bruce?"

A crackling response came back. "Wouldn't like to do this speed for too long, but everythin' topside's dealing with the punishment you're givin' it. Sure as fuck, I wouldn't want to be inside that box."

The skipper grimaced, showing a row of uneven yellowing teeth. Although they weren't speaking on an open channel, it was an electronic signal and his paranoia was running rife. "Shut the fuck up, Bruce."

He slammed the mic back onto its bracket and almost broke the clip. Without a word, Luke opened the fake fishfinder and flipped another switch.

"What ya doin'?"

"Just checkin' on our customers."

Matt grunted. "They'll be fine, they're down at fifteen metres and the dampeners on the rig should keep things smooth."

"Still, it's worth a look."

Luke clipped back the door of a cabinet revealing a TV and used a remote to select the second auxiliary channel. The screen split into four grey views of what looked like a rather sparse dormitory. All the occupants appeared to be sleeping in their bunks.

Matt glanced at the image. "Told you so."

A few moments later he checked his watch again, along with the GPS coordinates. "Made it back with only eight minutes to spare. We'll have to get those fuckin' Indos to come closer next time. Don't see why we should take all the risk."

He wiped his face and was surprised to feel the sweat on his brow. "I'll keep motoring for another five before throttling down for the VMS ping."

Luke didn't respond. After twenty years of sailing with his brother, he knew the last comment was not for his benefit. Matt often talked to himself when he was stressed. Luke switched off the TV and closed the cabinet, before leaning up against the chart table. He could do with another joint, but couldn't risk his brother's wrath if he got too stoned. He tried to relax by thinking of the money they'd make if they pulled this off. Although his brother would never admit it, he knew this was the last roll of the dice. The fishing industry had turned to shit, and he had seen the books before Matt paid off the accountant. If they didn't bring in some serious cash soon, they'd lose the boat.

The easing engine tone interrupted his thoughts as Matt pulled back on the throttle. "Right, Luke. Cut the auxiliaries, don't want that thing gaining on us."

"Sure."

"I'd hate to think what sonar signature those motors send out. Don't know of many trawl nets that sound like those goddam things humming along. We'll only use their extra power between net shots and when we're sure the coast is clear."

"Cool."

Luke flipped the relevant switches inside the fishfinder and looked at the red button. "You think we'll ever use the kill switch, Matt?"

The boat was now chugging at four knots and Matt relaxed a little. He turned to his brother and studied his face for a moment before answering. "I fuckin' hope not, it'll cost a fortune. But that said, if the need arises, don't ever think I won't do it. I'm not letting either of us go to the slammer for the fuckers in that can."

Luke stared back and nodded. "Me neither."

"Right. Now we've got that sorted out, let's plot a believable trawling pattern for the eyes in the sky. It'll take at least three days to reach Mornington from here."

9

HUNTED

It was eight in the morning and I was re-reading the online news article about the croc attack, while sipping my second cup of coffee. A picture of Charlie's beaming face was pride of place, shown holding his kitchen utensil with the banner headline "Crocodile Roll… in' Pin".

The bold text at the start read:

> ***Armed only with a small wooden rolling pin, Police Liaison Officer Charlie Parker jumped off a jetty to take on a five metre monster croc when it grabbed a local boy playing in the water near the island's boat ramp.***

I scrolled down to where there was a school photograph of Zac. He had been flown over to Townsville Base Hospital and the article reported him in a critical condition, but I knew from my sources he was out of theatre and doing well. When I first scanned the story, I'd been glad to discover the incomplete list of acknowledgements. The Mornington Island staff were mentioned, along with the Royal Flying Doctor Service and even the surgeons in Townville. However, there was no recognition of the ambo who fished the boy out of the sea and hauled his broken body to the A&E. It was a relief, as I'd asked all those involved not to mention my role. After all, I came here to avoid the media spotlight, and I didn't want my notoriety overshadowing Charlie's heroics.

With the story fresh in my mind, I decided to take a trip down to the jetty to view once again the scene of the action and see if I could spot the infamous reptile. It had become a bit of an island pastime now that Gununa was home to a monster croc.

I walked over to the station and found my newly acquired valet polishing the emergency lights on the roof of one of the Troopies. "Mornin' Paul. OK if I take the other one for a spin?"

He stood up and grinned. "Just as long as you don't get it too dirty, Jono. I haven't cleaned it yet."

I returned his smile and gave him a salute. "Yessir. I was going to drive it on the beach and throw a few donuts in the shallows before doing some off-road bush-bashing. Shouldn't get too messy."

I ducked to avoid the polishing rag thrown my way, before jumping in the cab and driving off. As I approached the jetty, I slowed to see what had drawn the attention of a small crowd over by the boat ramp. A man was winching a large metal cage off the back of a beat-up ute and was loading it onto the deck of a fishing boat.

I parked the Troopie and walked over to join the group of onlookers. The man turned out to be Oscar Fyans, a retired fisherman who lived on the outskirts of town. For the most part, he kept himself to himself. The few times I'd met him, he'd reminded me of Captain Quint, the shark catcher from *Jaws*. He even had the seventies facial hair and grumpy attitude to match. I'd never seen him wearing sunnies, and his tanned face had more creases than a dingo's scrotum. It was always good fun winding him up.

"You're going to need a bigger cage, Oz. The croc I saw will have to bend up double to fit in that."

He looked up to see who had spoken, then turned back to deal with the cage. "Tell you what, stretcher monkey, I'll work on catching the croc and you stick to bandages and slings."

I smiled at his cheap shot. "Here's hoping the croc takes your bait better than I do."

"I'm the one holding the Crocodile Management Authority for your problem animal, so you better hope I catch it. Otherwise, the next patient it provides may not be so lucky as that boy."

I moved in closer and helped guide the cage onto his boat. "Seriously, Oz, d'you think it's still hanging around this end of the island?"

He pulled the cage towards himself, then released the winch so it clattered onto the deck. "Crocs aren't stupid. They know when they're onto a good thing. That one will've been scoping out the jetty for days, waiting for someone to slip up. Y'see, they're ambush predators. What's more, they can wait a long time between feeds."

He turned around and looked out to sea. "I don't doubt he's watching us now."

My own eyes followed his gaze, but Oz seemed to drift off into his own thoughts and I stood there not knowing what to say. The sound of my mobile ringing disturbed the awkward moment. "Sorry Oz, got to take this. Anyway, best of luck with the hunt."

"Don't need luck."

"Right."

I walked away from the others on the boat ramp as I checked the screen. "Hi, Gee. What's happenin'?"

"G'day Jono. You have anything to do with that croc attack up there on Mornington? Didn't see your name in the papers."

"That's the way I like it these days. It was one hell of a big bastard, I saw the whole thing, but I'm sure you didn't call me to talk about crocs."

"True. Got some info on Plan Sea I thought you might want to hear."

"Go on."

"It would appear that Boardie sailed almost due east, with the first stop being Port Moselle, Noumea, in New Caledonia. He remained there for four weeks, the marina's maximum stay for foreign yachts, and then left the country. A few weeks later the yacht stopped at Rabaul in Papua New Guinea and after that Kendari in South East Sulawesi, Indonesia."

He paused, leaving me to finish his findings. "And then he disappeared?"

"Well, we know he made it to Indonesia, but over there, if you have enough money and find the right official, anything's possible."

"He's probably re-registered the vessel as Plan Dee."

"Don't joke. I'm sure that's what he did, and no doubt the new name'll be some sort of twisted pun, but it could be anything. It's the proverbial needle in the haystack."

I sighed. "What's the Indonesian word for needle? Maybe it's worth searching for a yacht with that name."

"Look, we'll find him. This lead may have dried up, but I've also been following the money. He had a substantial bank account in his fictional doctor's name, and it's still active. Only problem is that it's in Zurich."

"Switzerland? Shit."

"Interpol is on to it, but as everyone knows, their jurisdiction is limited in the world's banking capital."

"Right."

"Don't give up. I'm still hunting the bastard."

"I know. And thanks Gee."

As I closed the call, there was a rev of a diesel engine behind me. I turned to see Oz's boat easing away from the jetty, embarking on the hunt for the other monster in my life.

I sat among a group of locals for about an hour with my legs dangling off the jetty. We chatted and laughed about nothing in particular as we passed around an old pair of binoculars, taking turns to scan the water for a view of the crocodile. No one saw anything suspicious, but there were plenty of places for it to hide.

All along the adjacent island's edge, the verdant green foliage of the fringing mangroves folded into the calm waters, blurring the boundary between land and sea. Where patches of sand had been exposed by the tide, the aerial roots of the trees littered the ground with their gnarled finger-like projections, so that the shore resembled an expansive bed of nails.

Old Pete spoke as he handed me the binoculars for the umpteenth time. "So, Jono, as Charlie's not 'ere, what ya gonna name your croc?"

"You guys name them?"

"Only the big ones, eh."

I thought for a moment as I scanned the opposite shoreline. "Seeing as Charlie hit it with a rolling pin, it has to be Punch or Judy, don't you think?"

There were grins and generalised nodding, but Pete shook his head. "Can't be Judy."

"Why not?"

"Who the fuck's gonna be scared of a croc named Judy?"

"Good point. Punch it is then."

After another half hour there was still no sign of Punch and the midday heat got the better of me, so I returned to the aircon of my donga. An early light lunch was followed by the inevitable siesta, but the work's phone woke me at 2:30 PM.

"Mm, yer?"

"Wakey-wakey sleepy head, you've got an aggressive seventy-four-year-old woman to deal with at the APH. Proceed with caution."

"Right." I yawned down the phone. "On my way."

The Aged Person's Home was the island's only elderly-care facility and was about a minute's drive away. It was one of my regular call-out creators, and the jobs could be wide and varied. Although the corridors harboured the faint smell of stale urine that blights most nursing homes, the rooms were clean and had some of the best views I've seen from any government building. Set high, right on the beachfront, the prime location provided uninterrupted panoramic vistas over the sweeping Appel Channel and Denham Island beyond.

I pulled up the Troopie outside the entrance and the concerned-looking manager came out to meet me.

"Hi Margery, what's up?"

"Oh, Jono, I really don't know. It's Naomi, she's always been such a timid soul. She started acting weird this morning and now she's become violent and screaming all sorts of obscenities."

"What drugs does she take?"

"I'm not sure. The nurse'll know, but I'll print out a copy of her information sheet. Ellen here will show you to her room. I think you might have to sedate her."

"Have you guys given her anything?"

"We can't get anywhere near her."

I collected my bags and threw them on the stretcher, before following along behind Ellen through the maze of passageways.

It's one of the unerring laws of prehospital medicine: patients are always either on the top floor, or in the room furthest from the entrance. As we approached, I could hear the screaming and the sound of smashing ceramics. A young woman in a nursing uniform was standing next to the door, holding it closed. Her golden-brown skin contrasted with her crisp light-coloured dress, gleaming teeth and the whites of her wide-staring eyes. She wore her dark hair pulled back tight against her scalp and large gold loops dangled from her earlobes. She looked as if modelling would've been a better career choice than attending to the elderly.

"G'day, I'm Jono. What did you say to upset her?"

"Nothing. I've never seen her like this before."

"Hey, look on the bright side. At least it's plates and not shit she's throwing around."

Ellen laughed, and the girl gave me a horrified look. I grinned at her. "You must be new to working in a nursing home."

She nodded and moved back from the door.

"What's the old dear's name?"

"Naomi."

"Oh yes, that's right."

I knocked and the reply came back muffled. "Wha'?"

"Hello, my name's Jono, can I come in?"

"Suit y'self, ya fucka."

I shrugged and opened the door. As I peered in, the sight of a demure-looking woman sitting on the edge of a tidy bed greeted me. She was wearing a yellow and green floral dress with a white collar and a matching headband held back her wavy grey hair. Despite the cool of the room, beads of sweat covered her creased black face, and she was using a small lacy handkerchief to mop her brow.

"How're you feeling, Naomi?"

"Now dere's a stupid fuckin' question. Get da fuck outta ma room!"

She grabbed a tumbler from her bedside table and hurled it in my direction, just as I ducked and swung the door behind me. The glass shattered on the wall in an explosion of pieces, most of which clattered against the closing door.

I was checking my uniform for shards when Margery came bustling towards us, holding out a few sheets of paper. "Oh dear, oh dear. This is so unlike her. Here's everything we have on record. She's only been here a few months and doesn't take many medications. She's pretty self-sufficient, even organises her own insulin."

I stared at her, then turned to the nurse. "Insulin?"

"Yes. She keeps it in the fridge in her room."

"Right. I'm going to work under the assumption she's taken too much and she's having a hypo."

"Really? I thought they passed out."

"Eventually. But low blood sugar can change your behaviour..."

There was a scream from behind the door. "Fuck off ya cunts!"

I pointed towards the sound. "... just like that."

Margery looked aghast. "So what do we do?"

"I guess it depends on how strong you're feeling. There's one frail old lady and four of us."

The look on the three female faces in front of me answered my question, and I took out my mobile. "On the other hand, I can always phone a friend."

I was relieved to hear the other end pick up after a couple of rings. "Hey Charlie, you up to much?"

"I'm over at the youth club getting ready for footy training this evening. What's up?"

"I could use your muscles for about fifteen minutes over at the APH."

"You've got me intrigued, eh. I'll be there in a minute or two."

Margery walked back to the entrance to guide him in while I prepped my cannulation equipment, a bag of ten per cent glucose and a syringe loaded with the sedative midazolam. As I worked, there was a steady torrent of abuse coming from the room.

Everything was ready just as Margery returned with Charlie in tow.

"Hey, hey. Look who it is, Crocodile Dun-Don't."

"Yer, yer, you're goin' to tire of that one soon enough, eh. What's the problem, Jono?"

"Well, I've got a little old lady in there who's acting crazy. She's probably having a hypo and I need some extra muscle to hold her down while I check her blood sugar and give her some glucose."

He looked at the four of us standing there and furrowed his brow. "A little old lady?"

But his grin was short-lived as another explosion rattled the door and Naomi screamed at the top of her lungs. "Fuck off you bunch of cock-sucking cunt-fuckers!"

I shrugged and he nodded his appreciation. "So what's the plan?"

"OK, she's sitting in there on the left side of her bed, so I'll go in and talk to her. If I try and keep her focus on me, you can slip in and grab her from behind. If you can hold her arms and pin her face downwards on the bed with her head over the side, it'll stop her from spitting at us. Then one of these three can come in and lie across her legs, which'll allow me to cannulate her foot."

The nurse was open-mouthed. "Her foot?"

I shrugged. "People can't move their feet as easily as their hands. Anyway, from there I can give her either glucose or a sedative."

Charlie rubbed his chin. "OK, sounds good. Let's do it."

I turned to the three women who were looking at each other and pointed to the young nurse. "I'm guessing it's going to be you on the legs?"

She looked flustered. "Why?"

"Got to learn this stuff some time."

I smiled at her, gave a knock on the door and walked into the breach. As I entered, Naomi appeared to be moving things around her bedside cabinet, but the only item left was a large crystal ashtray.

"Hi Naomi, it's me again. Can we have a talk? I think your blood sugars are a bit low."

She turned to me as Charlie slipped into the room. "Thought I told ya ta fuck off."

But as he went to grab her, everything went to shit. Her eyes snapped in his direction and she grabbed the ashtray, swinging it in a wide arc towards him. Without thinking, I launched myself at her to stop the attack and, in an instant, she changed the trajectory of her swing. The next thing I saw was a cloud of stars as the crystal ornament connected with the side of my head. "Ah fuck."

"Fuck off ya cunts."

"Shit, you OK, Jono?"

"Grab her, Charlie."

Charlie bundled her up on the bed and called for the nurse, who came running in and held down the old woman's flailing legs. I just stood there holding my head, waiting for the wave of nausea to pass.

After a minute of wrestling with the screaming Naomi, the nurse looked up. "Are you going to do something?"

Her question brought me back to my senses, and I looked down at the three of them squirming around on the bed. “Right. What was the plan again?”

“Cannulate her foot. What’s wrong with you? Oh shit, what happened to your head?”

“I didn’t duck. I’ll be fine. Let’s get this show on the road.”

I took one of her shoes off and was glad to find a decent vein, which I managed to cannulate despite my developing headache. Her blood sugar came back as ‘Lo’, so I attached the bag of glucose and started pushing the contents through the line.

After a few seconds, she stopped struggling, and I had my two bouncers release their grip. “You OK, Naomi?”

She didn’t respond, but after a minute she rolled over as if waking from a long sleep. Sitting up with her back against the headboard, she eyed the three of us with suspicion and confusion. I was still squeezing the glucose when she spoke in an altogether different voice. “Who’re yous people an’ why’s ya in ma room, eh?”

“My name’s Jono. I think you might’ve taken too much insulin this morning.”

She slapped her hand to her forehead and scrunched up her eyes. “Oh, no! I’s had anudda hypo ain’t I, mista.”

I waggled the glucose bag at her. “Yep.”

“I’s hopes I din’t hurt no one, eh. Dem says I’s act like da devil ’imself.”

“Well, let’s say you weren’t as you are now.”

She pointed to my face. “Whats ’appened to ya head?” But before I answered, she put her other hand to her mouth. “Oh no way, it was me, was n’ it, mista. I’s so sorry, eh.”

“Don’t worry, I’ve had worse.”

Charlie joined in. “He has. Only last week gravity assaulted him. You've evened up his looks." Then his grin faded. "Er Jono, do you realise you're bleeding?"

I put my hand to my head and touched the developing egg. My gloved fingertips came away with blood on them. "Oh. If you'll excuse me, Naomi, I'd better sort this out."

She bobbed her head, eyes full of concern. "Yer, yer, ya go sort yaself, mista. I's so sorry, eh."

I passed the remains of the glucose bag to the nurse. "Could you check her blood glucose and keep pushing this if it's below four?"

"Sure."

There was a crunch of glass behind me as the two other women entered the room and I turned to look their way. Margery's mouth fell open. "What happened to your head?"

"Well, there was a flaw in my plan. Maybe you should confiscate Naomi's ashtray. Anyway, I'm going to use the en suite to patch myself up."

I grabbed a few items from my response bag and walked into the little adjoining bathroom, flipping on a light to check my head in the mirror. There was a sizeable bump on my left temple, centred around a small cut that was oozing blood. A red trail led down the side of my face, along my jaw, then down my neck to my collar. I'd thought it was a runnel of sweat.

I moistened some gauze with the tap water and started cleaning my skin, before using a new piece to apply pressure to the wound. I had picked up some steristips when the nurse walked in.

"Here, give me those."

"It's OK. I can do it."

"I don't doubt that, but it'll be easier if I do it. Come on, sit down."

I did as instructed and sat on the closed toilet seat. "Why

are nurses always so bossy, even new ones?"

"It's in our basic training. Here, now stay still."

She pulled the wound together with the sticky strips and pressed them in place with the gauze.

"Ow. And rough."

Her eyes twinkled and her smile revealed perfect pearly white teeth.

"Don't be such a baby."

She then set about covering the wound with a non-stick dressing, and I had nowhere else to look other than her uniform-covered breasts. I thought we'd better get acquainted. "By the way, you haven't mentioned your name."

"Jan. Now stay still."

"Really? I've got a friend in Brisbane called Jan. She's another ambo."

"Is that a friend, or a friend?" She emphasised the last word.

I hesitated as I thought about my old crewmate. "Just a friend. But either way, I'm not interested at the moment. I've... I've recently lost my fiancée."

"Lost her?"

The words still stuck in my throat and I was surprised how I'd let myself get this deep into a conversation with a complete stranger. "She... she was murdered."

The nurse stood back and looked at me. "Oh shit, you're *that* ambo!"

"Am I so infamous?"

"Sorry, I... the video of you saving the homeless man went viral. Everyone's seen it. You're a hero."

I snorted a laugh. "Not at all. Far from it. The only hero 'round here is my mate, Charlie. He was the one who battled a croc to save that kid the other day. Anyway, what's the story with Naomi?"

"Oh, yes, her blood's now six, so I've arranged for her to have something to eat. If you're happy, I'll take out the cannula and she can stay here. I don't think there's any point in her going to the hospital. Needless to say, I'll be managing her insulin from now on."

"Good idea. Have you finished with my head?"

"All done. Should match the one on the other side in a few days. Do you make a habit of this sort of thing?"

"I try not to. And thanks for patching me up."

"No worries."

I walked out to find Naomi sitting on her bed sipping a cup of tea and Ellen brushing up debris from the carpet. Charlie was standing in the doorway, nodding with his head for me to follow. "Hey, Jono. I've got to go."

"Thanks for your help Charlie, I'll see you out."

Once in the corridor, we moved away from the door. "What's up?"

He looked back to the room over my shoulder. "You know who your patient is, don't you?"

I shrugged. "Naomi?"

"Mrs Gibson."

"C'mon, you know I'm crap with names."

He lowered his voice to a whisper. "Dwayne Gibson?"

I looked blank, so he nodded his head towards the door. "That's Mr Wendal's mum."

"Oh shit. She's still alive? I presumed his relies would be dead by now."

"I think he's only in his fifties. Probably looks older from the way he's lived for the past twenty years, eh."

"Shit. Well, thanks for the info, I'd better get back in there. And thanks once again for the help, Charlie."

He walked off down the corridor, raising his hand in a

wave. "No worries, mate. It was worth it just to see you being belted by an oldie."

"You're all heart."

I returned to the room to the fading sound of his booming laughter and sat in a chair opposite my patient. "Right. How're you feeling now, Naomi?"

"Fine. I's so sorry for hurtin' ya head, eh mista."

"Don't worry. Where there's no sense, there's no feeling. I'll be fine. Jan here has done a great job of patching me up. Now, are you happy to stay here today?"

"Yes. I's not gonna no 'ospital, if dat's what ya mean, eh."

"Fine. OK, I'll need some details for my paperwork and then I'll be on my way. Do you have any medical problems other than your diabetes, like asthma or epilepsy?"

"No, not really, eh." She shrugged. "Just gettin' too old ta live on ma own."

"How's your ticker doing?"

She looked out the window. "Oh... dat was broke many years ago, eh, but da doc's say der's nuffin' wrong wid it."

Knowing the source of her heartache left me lost for words, but she read my expression as curiosity rather than consternation and sighed. "Oh, yous would'na know. Yous not from round 'ere, eh. Ma only child was accused of summat he did'na do and left da islan' years ago. I's sent people out lookin' fors him. Dey hunted high 'n' low, never found him, eh. An' he's never returned. He's probably deads now, not knowin' he's innocent."

Her eyes welled up with tears that trickled down her face and she wiped them with the back of her hand. "Sorry, eh mista. Dunna knows why I's tellin' you, eh. Not like yous can fix a broken heart."

I put down my note pad and held her hand. "I'm a paramedic. Fixing hearts is my speciality."

10

TLA

Matt and Luke were in the wheelhouse, while Bruce was leaning against the sorting table on the lower deck. The net was deployed and they were trawling at four knots. However, they were all staring at one thing - the fisheries patrol boat that was less than a kilometre away on their starboard side. About two hours ago a dot had appeared on the radar, which changed direction and had been shadowing their course ever since. So far, they seemed happy to observe from a distance, but the tension on the trawler was as taut as the hawsers towing the container.

"Perhaps they'll leave, they must know our licence is fuckin' good for what we're doing."

Matt took off his sunnies and licked the salt spray off his polarised lenses before replacing them. He did not share his brother's optimism.

As if to confirm his fears, the VHF radio sprang into life, causing Luke to flinch. "Fishing Vessel, Lady Jane, this is Boating Patrol. Please cease trawling operations and prepare to be boarded."

"What the fuck! They must be on to us."

Luke stood and made a move to the old fishfinder.

Matt spat out a command between clenched teeth. "Stand. Still. Now."

The low staccato tone of his voice made the statement all the more venomous, and his brother froze in his tracks.

"Don't make any quick movements, they can see us through binoculars from that distance. We've no reason to panic. That's what they're looking for, people rushing around when they make that first call."

He picked up the VHF mic and depressed the transmit button. "Boating Patrol, this is the Lady Jane. We still have an hour left on this shot. Can you bide your time? We are trying to run a business here."

There was a delay in their response and Luke stared at his brother with his eyes wide open. "We're on a schedule here, Lady Jane. You've thirty minutes to have your nets up and be ready for an inspection."

"Roger that Boating Patrol; we'll see what we can do."

Matt turned to Luke and smiled, exuding a calm that was only skin deep. "Stop worrying Luke, they're just bored. There's no other vessel for miles around and they've no doubt got a quota of fishermen to fuck with. They want to come on board and strut their stuff, show us who's boss and then they'll fuck off. You need to chill."

Luke looked anything but chilled. There was a slight tremor to his hands and his eyes were darting about as if he was on crack.

"Look, go smoke one of your joints while I delay them, but flush the rest of your stash down the head. And make sure Bruce does the same. I don't want this whole operation rolled because of some petty drug bust."

Luke took his sweat-soiled baseball cap off and rubbed his

greasy black hair. He replaced it, nodded at Matt and made his way down to the deck where Bruce was loitering.

Matt tapped his hand on the wheel and stared at the patrol boat. He could ill-afford the time for his crew to get stoned, but they needed something to calm their nerves. He checked the depth sounder: forty metres. As they hauled the net, he would slow and flood the ballast tanks to drop the rig to thirty-five and move it below the boat. That would mean the hawsers and umbilical would be almost vertical as they left the stern. They were hidden below the waterline, but he didn't want any chance of them being seen. He had already sunk the container from its cruising depth of nine metres to twenty as soon as the radar revealed a blip.

He pulled out a dive table from a drawer and inspected the numbers on the plastic sheet. They had about ten minutes at that depth before they would need a decompression stop. He shrugged. As long as he raised them back slowly to nine, they should be fine. Another day at that depth would give them plenty of time to de-gas. The main issue was the compressor. If that fired up while the filth was on board, they'd be snooping into everything, so he'd switch it off once they reached the holding depth. It might get stuffy down there, but his cargo would have to cope.

He looked at his watch and whistled down to Luke and Bruce. "Your time's up. Start bringing in the net. Don't want to piss 'em off too much."

The two men returned to the deck, a little more relaxed, and began winching the net. As soon as it was up, Luke hooked the suspended cod end and swung it over the sorting table before releasing the contents. A small collection of prawns fell out along with a large amount of by-catch, including sponges, rock, fish and a rather angry looking sea snake.

Luke turned to Bruce. "Don't remember loading the net with that one."

They both looked at each other and started giggling, while the snake writhed about among the catch, unimpressed by its treatment. As the net was only a decoy, they had caught the prawns and those in the ship's hold before the rendezvous with the Indonesians.

Matt called down from the bridge. "Can one of you two clowns get rid of that fuckin' snake and sort the catch? At least look as if you know what you're doing; they've started coming over."

Bruce gave a look of disgust. "That's gonna be your job, you know I can't stand snakes."

Luke shrugged. "Guess you're lucky you've got such a small cock."

"Fuck off."

Luke laughed and reached into the sorting table with a gloved hand, picking up the snake and lifting it into the air. He moved towards Bruce, who retreated to the stern. "Keep away, you fucker."

The reptile opened its mouth wide and made a low rasping sound, as it tried to curl its body back up to Luke's hand. Realising the game was up, he walked over to the gunwale and dropped it overboard.

"You'd think it'd be more grateful that I didn't cut its ugly head off."

"Do that again and I'll cut your fuckin' ugly head off."

The bump of the patrol boat against the trawler interrupted their banter. The Boating Patrol officers tied mooring lines to the available cleats, and two of them swung themselves up onto the deck. The third remained at the helm of their vessel.

Matt lit a large cigar and leant against the railing to the

side of the bridge. Without moving, he called down from his vantage point. "G'day. You able to make this quick?"

The two uniformed officers were dressed in smart light-blue shirts and darker blue pants, and both were wearing blue baseball caps with dark sunglasses. They looked like police, with insignia on their epaulettes and badges, but they had no guns. Unlike Matt, of course, whose pistol was resting out of sight, just inside the bridge door.

"Oh, you know the drill, we need to check your gear and see what you're catching. Won't take much of your time."

Matt took a pull on the cigar and eased the smoke out so that it circled round his head. "You better not, we've got work to do. Mind if my boys carry on sorting the catch?"

"By all means, but I'd appreciate if one of them could show me the hold, while my colleague checks your mesh size."

Matt sucked in another mouthful of smoke and let it seep out before nodding towards Luke. His brother acknowledged the instruction, then addressed the officer. "C'mon. This way."

The two of them disappeared from view and the other patrol officer began checking the net with a set of callipers, while Bruce started picking out prawns from the sorting table.

Matt stayed where he was. Close to his gun and the old fishfinder. He stole a glance at his watch. The rig had already been down at depth for over ten minutes. Just then, his heart rate cranked up a notch as he noticed an inconspicuous light flashing on the dashboard. Someone in the tin can had tripped the emergency button.

He chewed on his cigar. Well, the stupid fuckers would have to wait. He looked out to sea and the passage of a solitary gannet drew his eyes as it flew low over the waves. The bird kept going straight, as if on a mission, until the glare off the water made him blink and he could no longer make out its shape. He smiled to himself. It wasn't the first time he envied their freedom.

More time passed before Luke returned on deck with the Boating Patrol officer. They seemed to be having a friendly chat, and Matt gritted his teeth. Their quarter-million-dollar cargo could be drowning or suffocating to death, and his brother was chewing the fat with the filth.

He controlled his anger and let out a grumble, "Everythin' in order, officer?"

"Yes, all good. But I have to say you haven't got much to show for over a week's trawling. You've got your TEDs fitted, but have you thought of using other BRDs? It would speed up your sort time."

Matt leaned forward onto the adjacent railing and spoke with the cigar still clenched between his teeth. "I beg your pardon, I'm not one for TLAs."

"TLAs?"

"Three letter acronyms. Now have you finished your inspection?"

The patrol officer glanced at his colleague, who nodded. "Er... yes."

"Well, you'd better GLF, or your LWA will be FFF."

He looked confused.

"GLF? Go Like Fuck. LWA? Lilly White Arse. FFF? Fuckin' Fish Food. Now get the fuck off my boat."

For a moment it appeared as if he was going to stand his ground and try to regain some authority with the skipper. Then the stark reality of being so far from anywhere with nothing to protect themselves kicked in.

He gave Matt a curt nod before turning and climbing onto the patrol boat. As he and his crewmate released the mooring lines, he called back. "Oh, and don't forget to note that sea snake in your log book."

"Already done."

The three of them watched as the other boat motored away, their wake churning a white trail that shimmered in the sunlight. When they had gone some distance, Luke climbed up to join his brother on the bridge. "Jesus, Matt, did you have to fuck with them so much?"

He took out his cigar and blew a smoke ring before grinning. "If I was nice to them, they'd have known something was up. Now switch on that monitor, while I fire up the compressor and start raising the rig back to cruising depth."

He stepped towards the old fishfinder and flipped open the cover, grabbing a small microphone and pressing the transmit button. "What the fuck's going on down there? What's your fuckin' emergency?"

11

PRESSURE

If the initial week had been bad, then the journey over the last couple of days had become unbearable. Ahmad Nasim lay in his bunk holding his head, trying to cope with the endless earache and recurring migraines. His parents had given up their life savings for this service, but he wished he could go back and confront the constant risk of Taliban reprisals. Anything had to be better than another minute of this torture.

A man's face appeared at the entrance to his bunk. Rashid Moradi smiled a welcome, stretching out his bushy moustache that was now accompanied by thick stubble on his normally clean-shaven chin. His receding hairline accentuated the round appearance of his face, while his swarthy complexion added further depth to his close-set eyes. "Hey Nasim, you good for English lesson, no?"

Nasim pried one eye open. "That depends, Rashid. Have you got any more of those white pills?"

"I tell you before, my friend. Too many not good. What wrong now?"

"Headache, earache." He groaned. "And I feel like shit."

Rashid's face disappeared and was back within a few minutes. Holding out his hand. "This. Eat two. They will help with... how you say... pressure?"

"Pressure?"

"Yes, pressure. Lot of water push down on us."

"What? You think we're underwater?"

"Yes, yes. Underwater, like... submarine, but not..."

He frowned in concentration, but he had to finish his sentence in Farsi. "This container we're in is not at a fixed pressure like a submarine. It keeps changing, depending on how deep we go. It's more like a diving bell. That's why your ears are hurting."

Nasim rolled over to look at him and continued the conversation in his friend's preferred language. "What makes you think we're underwater?"

He shrugged. "The motion. The cold. The condensation on the walls. The pressure fluctuations. The sounds." He shrugged again. "I thought it was obvious. We've been underwater ever since they moved us off what I can only guess was a container ship. Listen, hear that distant whirring sound?"

Nasim pointed to his ear. "I'm finding it difficult to hear you."

"Well, trust me, it's there. It's a boat's propellor. They're towing us in underwater to avoid detection. What you need to do, my friend, is keep clearing your ears, like this."

He demonstrated the same bizarre behaviour the woman on the plane had shown him. It felt months ago when all this craziness began. Nasim attempted to copy him, but Rashid stopped his hand before it reached his nose.

"Not now, my friend. Not now. Wait thirty minutes for my tablets to work, then have a go, but be very gentle. Your ears should clear, but rest now; I'll be back in a while for my

English lesson." He smiled and lowered himself from the opening.

Left alone, Nasim curled into a foetal position, as much as his cramped sleeping area would allow, and tried not to think about the tonnes of water above him.

He woke to the gentle shaking of his shoulder and saw Rashid smiling at him. "My tablets worked well, no?"

Nasim looked around his bunk and for the first time in days the movement of his head caused no pain. "Wow, what were they? That's the best sleep I've had in ages."

"It was a strong... How you say, to clear nose?"

"Decongestant?"

"Yes. Decongestant. That's it, with... opiate? You sleep for five hours."

"Really? Five hours? Well, I guess I needed it." He rubbed his face, yawned and pushed his arms against the ceiling of his bunk to stretch his muscles. "Right, I suppose we'd better start that lesson."

Rashid smiled and dropped from view, while Nasim dragged himself out of his bunk and climbed down to the floor. There he tied back the curtain that gave some privacy to the tiny bathroom and sat on the toilet seat, looking up at the rows of bunks. "So, how many students do I have today?"

Rashid had returned to his bunk, the entrance now framing his face. Six more faces smiled back at him, and the man in the bunk above his head called out. "I'm in too."

The only one not interested on this side of the container was the beautiful woman with the green eyes. She always kept herself to herself and for the most part stayed in her bunk until the lights dimmed to indicate night time. Then she would emerge when she thought everyone was asleep and perform a silent gruelling exercise routine. She scared Nasim, and he was glad he didn't have to interact with her now.

"Right, so what would you like me to explain?"

As he spoke, he poured himself a cup of water from the tap next to him.

Rashid grinned. "I not drink that, my friend. Only drink protein shakes."

Nasim looked in the clear fluid. "Why not? I know it tastes odd, but it's OK, isn't it?"

"Well, two day back..."

"Two days ago would be more correct."

"What? Oh, yes, yes. Two days ago I have suspicion..."

"I became suspicious."

"Right. And I drop colour tablet, you know, for teeth, in toilet."

"Colour tablet?"

"Yes... Show teeth not brushed good."

"Oh. I'm not sure, but I think they're called disclosing tablets. Why do you have them?"

"Back in Iran, I was dentist."

"I was 'a' dentist."

"Really, you too?"

"No. I was correcting your English. Anyway, what happened?"

"When?"

"The tablet in the toilet."

"Oh yes, next day water from tap slight pink colour."

"THE next day THE water from THE tap was... Oh shit, we're drinking our own urine!"

"Yes, yes. It is filter, but still."

"That's disgusting." He threw the contents of the cup into the sink. "How come the rest of you aren't surprised?"

Another man responded with a shrug. "He told us yesterday."

"What?"

"You asleep, my friend. This first time… Wait, listen."

They all went quiet, but after a while Nasim broke the silence. "What's wrong? I can't hear anything."

"Exact. No engine sound."

Suddenly Rashid screwed up his face and put a hand to his head. "All you, blow on your nose now, we going down fast!"

Pressure built in Nasim's head and he grabbed his nose, blowing hard to clear his ears, but the effects of the medication had worn off. Nothing he did would equalise the pressure. And the pain soon followed, radiating into his head. As the sensation intensified, a ringing sound started, and he looked around for the alarm, but all the other faces were just staring at him. He dropped to his knees, holding his head, and again tried to blow his nose, but the pain just got worse. He called out, but couldn't hear his own voice, and as he sucked in a breath, it seemed as if the air was getting thicker.

He started to hyperventilate, then there was a pop sensation in his head and the room spun. He closed his eyes, but the vertigo worsened, and he felt for the toilet, flipping the lid before vomiting in the bowl. A hand patted his back, but he brushed it aside.

After his stomach contents were spent, Nasim clawed at the floor, which appeared to be undulating. He somehow got enough purchase to launch himself at the wall and, once upright, reached and hit the emergency button. "Let me out! Let me out! Let me out!"

Even in his panic, he caught sight of a blurred movement in his peripheral vision, then an arm snaked around his neck. The limb was smooth and feminine, but was like steel as it tightened against both his carotids. He struggled, but his flailing arms and legs contacted nothing more solid than the viscous air his lungs were struggling to suck in. As the edges of his vision blackened, a quiet voice caressed his consciousness. "Don't worry, just relax. No need to fight, you'll be fine."

Then there was darkness.

Those who had left their bunks stared in disbelief at the limp body of their would-be English teacher, now held in the arms of the green-eyed woman. Rashid spoke first. "You kill him?"

"No. He's just knocked out. Look, see, he's still breathing. He might wake with a headache, but there'll be no lasting effect."

"How you do that?"

"You don't want to know."

In the silence that followed, the Iranian man held out his hand. "Er, my name Rashid. We have not introduce."

She laid Nasim's unconscious body on the floor and paused before accepting the proffered hand and making a slight bow. "Tshaarre."

They stood for a moment, not knowing what else to say. They were like enemy combatants sharing a cigarette in no-man's-land. It was a simple social gesture, but rather than breaking the ice, it only underlined their mutual distrust.

Tshaarre was the first to speak, pointing at Nasim. "Unless you all want to lift his body up there, one of you in the lower bunks will have to swap with him. I think if he's near the floor, it'll be safer for all of us. I have some sedatives I can use if he goes crazy again."

There was generalised nodding, and they set about rearranging the bunks, sliding the unconscious Nasim into his new sleeping space. Just as they finished, the intercom crackled into life. "What the fuck's going on down there? What's your fuckin' emergency?"

The woman walked over to face one of the cameras. “False alarm. A man panicked when you dropped us deep. He hit the button before I could stop him. I had to subdue him, but he’ll be fine.”

“Right. Well, make sure you keep a better fuckin’ handle on things down there if you ever want to see daylight again.”

12

SWEERS

"Holy crap, you're actually taking that thing out on the water? That old woman must've given you a serious head injury."

I turned around to see Albert standing at the front door of his donga, with his chest puffed out like a sunburnt cane toad.

"Mornin' Albert. Thought I deserved a short break off island, so I booked a few nights at Sweers."

"You sure that tinnie can make it that far?"

I continued to unfurl the tarp off my boat. "She's managed it before. This little beauty has a seventy-five-horsepower Mariner strapped to the back. She flies like shit off a shovel, just gotta make sure her fuel tanks are full."

"And that you don't meet your croc again."

"Ha. Like to see Punch catch up with me."

"Punch?"

"Big bastard crocs apparently get a nickname. Anyway, he hasn't been spotted since grabbing Zac. So far, all Oz has trapped are a few young pretenders. I'm guessing Punch has buggered off to the mainland."

"Still. I wouldn't want to be in a small boat like that if it came looking for lunch."

"Haven't you got something better to do?"

Albert yawned and stretched his arms, then looked around the yard. "Nope."

"Well, in that case, you can give me a hand getting her in the water."

He snorted. "Shit. Should have seen that coming."

"Thought you'd do anything to get me out of your hair for a few days."

"You've got a point. I'll go get the Troopie."

He strode off to the vehicle shed and left me shaking my head. By the time I'd loaded my dry bag, esky, fishing gear and safety equipment, Albert was reversing the ambulance towards the trailer. I hooked her up and we set off to the boat ramp.

Albert was the first to break the silence of the cab. "It's odd how I've come back to a pair of spotless ambulances. I find it hard to believe you've made it a priority to clean them for my return."

I gave him a sideways glance. "Cleanliness is next to godliness, Albert. While you were away, I found religion and I'm going to Sweers for a prayer meeting."

"You're so full of shit it just keeps flowing out of you, doesn't it? Is there any chance you'll ever give me a straight answer?"

I thought about his question. "Nope."

"Look, I know why you're going to Sweers. It's the closest island with an actual bar, and you've probably run out of your not-so-secret stash of rum. Do me a favour and don't get too pissed."

"I'm offended you'd think I'm so shallow. As to the state of the Troopies, there's a local lad, Paul, doing a two-month stint of community service. He'll be around each morning to clean them. Not sure what he got busted for, but I don't think he wants to talk about it. Either way, it's a win for us as he's doing a damn good job. Oh, could you pull over at the fuel station? I've got to fill up my tanks."

Once all four tanks were topped up, we drove the remaining short distance to the ramp and Albert reversed the trailer into the water. I then released the stays and my boat floated free of its harness. I jumped on board after Albert waded in knee-deep to hold the bow.

"Thanks for that, Albert. See, you love me really."

"Love to see the back of you, more like."

I revved my engine before engaging the prop. "Sorry Albert, didn't catch that. Have a wonderful time while I'm gone. I'll send you a postcard."

"Don't hurry back."

"Better get out of the water before Punch gives you a love bite."

I waved as I reversed away from the ramp, manoeuvring the boat around so I could drive out into the channel. But before setting off, I spotted Oz checking his trap and drove over to say hello.

"G'day Oz. Catch anything?"

He was now leaning against the wheelhouse of his boat, watching my approach with a glum expression. "S'pose you're here to offer me some advice."

"Well, I saw the bastard, and I wasn't joking when I said you'd need a bigger trap."

"I guess we'll see how this one does." He pointed to the partially submerged cage, which his boat had obscured from my view. "They sent it over on the barge, yest'dee. It's the largest they have. If he's still here, I'll catch him."

"That looks good. Hey Oz, you keep saying 'he'. Did we get it right with Punch and not Judy?"

"I heard that's the name goin' around. Yes. Big salties're always male. Was it a lucky guess?"

I shrugged. "Apparently Judy wasn't scary enough."

While talking, I looked in the trap to discover a huge piece of meat suspended from the ceiling. "Jesus, Oz, if that carcass doesn't attract it, nothing will. What was sacrificed to produce that?"

"Oh, they sent me over a load of feral pigs. Crocs love the stuff."

"Who doesn't like pork? Well, except firies. They say when cooked it smells like burnt bodies."

He raised his eyebrows and gave me a strange look. Then I remembered I wasn't talking to another paramedic. "Right, on that note, I'd better be off."

"Gettin' some fishin' in?"

"Yes, off to Sweers for a few nights."

The corners of his mouth curled up a fraction, but not enough to call it a smile. "Given up on beach drinking, have ya?"

His question surprised me. "Shit. Does everyone know about that?"

He pulled the peak of his cap down towards his eyes. "Not much happens on this island without someone finding out."

After leaving Oz to his crocodile hunting, I opened the throttle of my outboard and sent my sixteen-foot Easyrider skipping across the glass-calm waters of the channel. Last night, I'd checked the Bureau of Meteorology website. There was no rain forecast for the next few days, but squalls in this area were difficult to predict. I found it somewhat ironic that the BoM radar for the whole Gulf region stood on the ground behind my donga, but I would still look out the window to see what the clouds were doing.

Once the boat was up on the plane, with only the prop cutting through the waves, it felt so good to be out on the water again. The wind on my face. The freedom of the open sea. I tried to push the inevitable thoughts of Amber to the back of my mind, but gave up and imagined her standing next to me in the cockpit, her jet-black hair flying around her head, the sound of the engine and the roar of the wind almost drowning out her laughter. I had to smile to myself; at least I'd have some company for the journey.

As Denham Island passed behind me on the starboard side, I followed the lee of Mornington for a short while, before striking out on my compass bearing towards Sweers. I checked the satnav agreed with my direction and settled in for the ride. At the speed I was travelling, I'd make it in ninety minutes.

After about an hour, I pulled back on the throttle and came down off the plane. Mornington was so low-lying it had long since disappeared over the horizon, and I could see Bentinck Island in the distance. On a day like today, it would be a crime not to do a little deep-water fishing.

I baited a couple of lines and cast them off the stern, clicked the throttle into gear, and began trolling toward Sweers to try and snag a meal. The mid-morning sun beat down as I sought refuge under my boat's small canopy. Grabbing out a can of Coke from beneath the ice in the esky, I savoured the fizzy cold liquid as it rolled down my throat. The engine chugged like that for some time, and I relaxed in my swivel chair, waiting for a hit on the line. This was the life. No managers, no work hassles, no whinging patients, no serial killers. Just my boat, the ocean, and me.

"But how long would it be before you got bored?"

I turned to see Amber standing there in her black bikini,

breathtaking in her relaxed beauty. "Oh shit, I've fallen asleep, haven't I?"

"C'mon, answer the question."

I thought for a moment. "I reckon I could live on a boat for some time, if I had the funds to keep me going."

"But you'd strive for more. Hiding away here on an island is like being on a boat. Water all around with few ties to reality, but has it got you your happiness? Have you sorted out your head yet?"

"You were my happiness and you're gone. You'll always live on in my mind, in my thoughts, but it'll be a long while before I'm happy again."

"You need to let me go, Jon. This isn't healthy for you."

"What if I don't want to?"

She shook her head. "You need to stop wallowing in self-pity, you need to..."

Bang! There was a smash as something hit the boat, then an enormous set of scaly green jaws swung into view, grabbing Amber by the midriff and dragging her overboard. I yelled and leapt to the side, but all I could see was a swirling mass of bloodstained water. Suddenly her hand thrust up above the waves and I grabbed it, pulling with all my might. Then something gave, and I fell backwards onto the deck. When I sat up, I was horrified to find the bloody severed hand of my fiancée lying in my lap, her engagement ring twinkling in the sunlight.

My eyes shot open to discover I had slipped down in my seat, but I was still underneath the canopy, a ticking-whir sound coming from the stern. It took me a moment to realise it was one of my reels paying out line, so I pushed the nightmare to a dark corner of my mind, flicked the throttle into neutral and leapt across the deck to grab the rod.

Slowing the travel of the line, I began reeling in my prize. Fifteen minutes later I sat on the transom, tired but triumphant and admiring the huge long-fin tuna I'd landed. At least I had something impressive to present to the other fishers when I arrived at Sweers.

I looked up to check my location and was surprised to see that Bentinck Island was far closer than I expected. How long had I been asleep? I checked my watch. It couldn't have been too long. Had I left the motor in gear? No, it was definitely in neutral. I looked around and spotted some seaweed floating along at the same speed as the boat and realised I was sitting in a strong current flowing towards Bentinck. Sweet, the water movement had no doubt saved me some fuel.

I dumped my fish in the esky, having to leave its tail sticking out the side, and climbed back in the driver's seat. Opening up the throttle, I was on the plane in a matter of seconds, hammering my way over to Sweers.

The rest of the journey was uneventful, and I was soon pulling my boat up onto the golden sands of the Sweers beachfront, a little ways up from the resort's fleet of tinnies. The reflected sun shone off their aluminium hulls and I could see there were a few gaps in the lineup; some guests must still be out fishing.

I threw my anchor out high above the strandline, then grabbed my dry bag and esky and lugged them towards the resort. It had to be said that 'resort' was a bit of a grand name for the main eating area and collection of communal cabins dotted around the well-tended lawns. But what it lacked in facilities, it made up for in charm. Plus, it had the only licensed bar in the whole of the Wellesley Islands.

I lumbered up over the foreshore and onto the path towards the reception. A light breeze tempered the heat and played through the scattered palms, causing the fronds to sway and the leaflets to chatter together. The green feathery branchlets of the numerous casuarinas joined in with the rhythmic motion, and it felt like I was being treated to an arboreal welcome dance.

The manager, Pam Brookfield, came walking down the path to meet me. Her sun-tanned wrinkled face creased in a welcoming smile and she stood with her arms open. Her blonde curly hair looked like it had remained in the same style since the sixties, along with her choice of clothes.

"G'day Jono, you must've made good time. D'you bring me anything decent?"

"G'day, Pam. Can you use a long-fin to add to your menu?"

"Only if you get in the kitchen and give our chef a hand preparin' it."

I put down the esky, and she moved closer, giving me a big hug.

"Good to see you again, m'boy. You shouldn't be such a stranger; it's been a while since you were here last."

"Oh, 'bout three months. I do have to work, y'know."

"True. I guess you were involved with that boy the croc grabbed. What an awful business. D'you know how he's doing?"

"Still in Townsville, but he should make a full recovery. Although I can't imagine he'll want to swim again, at least in the sea. He was damn lucky Charlie was there with his rolling pin."

"That man's a legend. They'll have a statue of him before you know it. Anyway, let's get you settled in. I've got you in one of the two-bed cabins. We've a couple of big groups staying at the moment. They're pretty rowdy, so I thought if I put you on your own you can choose whether or not to join in."

"Thanks Pam, you're a star."

She gave me a smile. "Gotta look out for our ambos, never know when you'll need one. Hey, what the hell happened to your forehead? Looks as if you've been clamped in a vice."

"You wouldn't believe me if I told you. Let's say one of them's got something to do with a vice of mine."

She laughed. "C'mon vice-captain. Leave your esky there, I'll show you to your room."

The light from a street lamp threw my shadow on a wall as I crept along the pavement in the dead of night. Despite my quiet footfalls, I disturbed a restless fruit bat that dropped from its perch with a flapping 'whump whump' sound as its leathery wings made strong downthrusts to gain altitude. I could make out its dark shape against the night's sky as it squeaked its annoyance, before flying away to another tree.

I placed a hand out to steady my slow advance and the bricks of the wall felt cold. I wasn't sure why there was a need to be so stealthy, but I recognised the street and my heart was already thumping in my chest. I'd been here before. Just up ahead was the alley where I'd confronted Boardie and where he'd forced me to let him go in order to save Mr Wendal's life.

Although the night air was cool, I could feel sweat trickling down my neck and my Spidey senses were shrieking. I knew I should turn around, call the cops, or wait for backup. But my feet kept stepping, one foot in front of the other. My curiosity was stronger than my growing fear.

As I approached, I heard muffled noises coming from deep inside the alley. At first they were difficult to determine. Was it breathing, or was someone choking? But the closer I drew, the clearer they became. It was a woman's voice making the rhythmical throaty sounds of sexual pleasure.

I stopped in my tracks. What was I doing here? I'm not a voyeur. This was all wrong. I tried to turn back, but my body was drawn to the opening like a cow dragged into an abattoir. I stepped into the alley and the stench of rotting food from the garbage bin greeted me. The woman's grunting sounds were louder now. She appeared to be reaching a climax, and I was grateful to be blind to the scene, hidden by the alley's inky blackness.

Then, to my horror, my hand reached down to my utility belt and unclipped a flashlight. My mind screamed as I tried to stop my arm raising and my thumb from depressing the button. But it was all to no avail. There was a click and a cone of brilliant white light lit up the alley.

There, amongst all the filth, was the naked figure of a woman, kneeling astride the motionless body of an Aboriginal man whose trousers were below his knees. Her hips were thrusting down on his mutilated genitals, as she whipped around her long black hair in the throes of passion. With each push of her creamy white buttocks, a jet of red liquid spurted from a hole in the man's neck, spraying blood across the adjacent wall like a talentless macabre graffiti artist.

I tried to drop the torch. Tried to turn and run. Tried to scream. Just tried to close my eyes. But I could do nothing other than watch as she turned her head and smiled at me.

Somehow I found my voice and managed a croak. "Amber... no..."

She laughed. "Now will you leave me in peace?"

"But Amber... I still love you..."

"I'm dead, Jon. You have to move on. Go back to Brisbane. Restart your life. This man's still alive, and you know how to save him. Do that, and at least something good can come out of all this shit. Do that and I might stop haunting you."

With another smile, she turned to Mr Wendal and bent

down as if to give him a kiss. But then she put her mouth to his neck wound and when she looked back, blood was trickling from her chin.

"Carry on as you are and sooner or later you'll grow to hate me."

Then she spat out the mouthful of blood and as the liquid hit my face, I sat upright in bed. The sheets in my air-conditioned cabin were drenched in sweat.

13

PROBLEM

Two headlights disturbed the remote Mornington coastline, blinking three times in the darkness. Matt snorted his relief. "About fuckin' time."

He put down the binoculars he'd been using to scan the shore for the past hour and stepped outside the bridge, using his flashlight to acknowledge the signal. The south side of Mornington Island was a dark smudge in the distance, lying like a half-submerged crocodile on a moonless night.

"D'you see him? Did he give the OK?"

"Stop your worrying, Luke. It's all going to plan. The rig's about a metre down now. I'll leave it there until the boat arrives. Don't want any waves showin' it's there."

The rest of the journey had been uneventful and after arriving at the rendezvous point, he'd began the slow process of raising the container to the surface.

Luke's eyes darted back and forth, peering into the gloom. "Shit, d'you think someone's out there watchin' us?"

The older brother sighed. "Jesus, Luke, chill out."

He pointed to one of the screens in front of him. "See for

yourself, there's nothing on the radar other than that single blip there, which is our contact coming to meet us."

Luke peered at the monitor and after a while his shoulders relaxed a little. He walked over and sat on the map table, swinging his legs like a hyperactive schoolchild. Then he froze and his mouth fell open. "Oh shit. Look."

Matt looked at the radar, but there was still only one dot. "What?"

Luke's eyes were wide as he pointed to the small light on the dashboard that was flashing on and off.

"Ah fuck, what now? Switch on the TV and get the surveillance feed up."

Matt picked up the microphone, but waited for the video images before depressing the transmit button. The four grey pictures flickered into view and centre stage was the woman, Tshaarre, staring out of the screen with all the warmth of a shark looking at its next meal.

"What?"

"There's a problem. Not sure what's happening, but one man started scratching and now most of us feel like our skin's crawling with fleas. It spread quick, but I can't find the cause."

"Is that it? You called an emergency 'cos you're itchy? Could just be fuckin' bed mites."

She had her arms folded across her chest and as she spoke her hands scratched the skin of her upper arms. "No. The man who first started itching is now unconscious and two more have pissed themselves."

"Pissed themselves?"

"Yes. They say they can't feel their legs."

The sound of an approaching motor interrupted their conversation. Matt closed his eyes and shook his head. "Fuck."

He then pressed the mic's button. "I'll get back to you."

Luke looked aghast. "What's going on Matt?"

"Fuck knows. Could be some weird Asian parasite, or maybe it's from drinking their own piss. How the fuck should I know? Stay here and watch the screens while I go meet me old mate. He might have some idea of what to do."

He stormed out of the bridge and slammed the door before sliding down the stair rails and onto the deck. His feet landed with a thud as the other boat pulled alongside and Matt caught the line thrown to him. After he secured the vessel to the trawler, their new guest swung himself aboard.

Matt thrust out a hand in greeting. "Good to see you again, Oz. Hate to tell you this, but we've got a fuckin' problem."

14

RUNS

All up, I spent five nights on Sweers, though I was reluctant to sink more than a couple of stubbies in the evenings after that skinful-induced nightmare. Instead, I joined the other guests on their fishing trips, did a bit of bushwalking and enjoyed a relaxing break. As I waved goodbye to Pam, I felt quite positive for the first time in about a year. It helped that I'd come to some sort of decision about my future, and my future was in Brisbane. Perhaps I'd sorted out my head, or at least been forced to do so. Perhaps that nightmare had been my turning point.

The journey back was a little rougher and the slight swell meant I had to concentrate to stay on my bearing. The salt spray and the thumping of the hull into and over the waves was both exhilarating and tiring. By the time I made the lee of Mornington, my positive outlook had faded like a beach ball left in the sun. Albert had always given me so much shit about townies never lasting a full term on the island and now I was going to prove him right. The realisation I'd have to spend months with his smug 'I told you so' expression was taking its toll.

When I reached Gununa, I felt bruised and battered, and it wasn't just physical. As ever, Old Pete was sitting on the jetty, handline in the water. "Aft'noon, Jono. Yous been gone a whiles. Catch anythin' decent?"

"Got an esky full of snap-frozen fillets. Give me a hand off-loading and you can have a few."

He gave me a toothless grin. "Deal."

I looked around the carpark, but there was no sign of the Troopie. "Don't suppose you've seen Albert or Charlie? I sent them both a text to come meet me."

He'd reeled in his line and caught my painter, looping it over one of the wooden posts. "Nar. Fat chance you've got of dat, eh. They'lls be up at the footy match."

"Shit. Should've known. Guess I'll have to walk. D'you mind watching my boat while I go get the Troopie?"

He gave another grin. "Sure. But I's choose the fillets."

I laughed. "You drive a hard bargain, Pete."

I soon returned in one of the ambulances and with Pete's help had my boat out of the water and back outside my donga in no time. But then came the offload and clean up, after which I was shattered. There were still shouts coming from the footy field, but going there meant I'd have to face Albert. I looked at the setting sun disappearing from view and felt its fading colours reflected my ebbing resolve. That confrontation could wait until tomorrow.

I woke the next day feeling drained and anything but positive. There'd been no nightmares, but I'd hardly slept. Despite my fatigue, I decided a run might help and before long I was out pounding a dirt road, the metronomic thump of my joggers soothing my soul. Cycling used to be my therapy, but I hadn't been back on a bike since Mr Wendal...

Just the thought of his name was enough to send my mind to the edge of a spiraling, guilt-ridden wormhole, so I started sprinting. I ran faster and faster until my heart was thudding and the only thing I could think about was the searing pain in my lungs and muscles. My foot clipped a rock causing me to stumble, so I stopped in the shade of a large sprawling beach almond. Bent over double, my hands on my hips, I gulped in deep breaths, filling my chest with the warm morning air.

Holding out a hand, I leant against the rough sturdy trunk of the tree. The canopy of waxy emerald leaves were in stark contrast to the nearby bushes and I was glad of the respite from the wakening sun. The track stretched out ahead of me and off in the distance were the aquamarine waters of the Gulf, with birds dotting the sky like the settling particles in a snow globe. It was a glorious morning.

Letting out a laugh, I shook my head. What was I worried about? As Amber had graphically demonstrated, Mr Wendal was one wormhole I could plug. In fact, nothing was stopping me from flying to Brissie in my next six days off and dragging his scruffy arse back to see his mum. Then at least that mental slate could be wiped clean.

I nodded to myself. Whatever it cost to bring him home, it would be a darn sight cheaper than years of psychotherapy, and this way more people would benefit. I took a slug from my water bottle, turned around and started jogging into town.

Once again, I looked at the office clock and back at the empty chair in front of me. It was 12:05 PM and no Albert. The first time I'd turned up early to one of his meetings and the pompous bastard was late. I wondered if he was winding me up. After checking my work emails and twiddling my thumbs for another fifteen minutes, I wandered into the hospital.

"G'day Gloria, you seen Albert about?"

She looked up from her desk, a little startled. "Oh, hey Jono." She frowned and shook her head. "No, not since yesterday. He was going on about some paperwork regarding an RFDS transfer. I'll have to admit, I switched off. How were your days away, do anything nice?"

"Yes, thanks, I did. Been fishing over at Sweers Resort."

"All right for some. D'you make up for that sailfish?"

"No such luck. Charlie's got a lot to answer for. Anyway, I'd better find my boss, you know how he likes his handover meetings."

"Surprised you're chasing him for one of those."

I shrugged. "It's simpler to get it over with. Catch ya later."

With both Troopies parked in their shelter, the only place left was his donga, but Albert never stayed there on a workday. I walked to his demountable and rapped my knuckles on the screen door. "Albert?"

I stood there listening, but the only sound came from the chirping cicadas. I knocked again, this time louder. "Albert, are you in there?"

There was a muffled groan from the bedroom, followed by padding steps stumbling towards the entrance. Then the door opened to reveal Albert. Well, someone who resembled Albert. His tanned skin was pale, his eyes bloodshot, and his free hand had a slight shake as he held onto the door with the other.

"Jesus, Albert, you look like shit. Have you been on the piss?"

"No, of course not! I've got food poisoning. It must have

been from the barbecue after the footy yesterday. Whatever I ate had me up all night. I don't know which end to point at the dunnie."

"You want me to call an ambulance?"

"Hilarious. Just cover for me today, I'm hoping it'll work its way through."

"Did you want any anti-emetics, or a bag of fluid?"

"What? And have you cannulate me seventeen times? No thanks."

"Oh, c'mon. I'd make sure I got a line in after at least the tenth go. Seriously, do you need anything?"

"No. Other than about twelve hours sleep without one of my sluice gates opening."

I nodded and gave a sigh. "I did have something to discuss with you today, it was about my future here."

Albert's face took on a pained expression, as if he was trying to open a beer bottle with his anal sphincter. "It'll have to wait. Gotta go!"

He slammed the door, and I heard his stomping footsteps recede away, then the sound of a splash, followed by the moan of an injured animal. "Oh nooo!"

I could have offered my assistance. I could have helped my colleague in his hour of need. With all things considered, my role is within a caring profession. But I deemed mopping up Albert's shit above and beyond the call of duty. So I crept away from his door before jumping in a Troopie and going for a long drive to nowhere in particular.

I checked on Albert later that arvo, but he was just grumpy because I'd disturbed him, so after that I left him to sleep it off. It was a pretty slow day, and I was clearing up a reef-fish supper when my personal phone rang with a number marked 'private'.

"Y'ello?"

"Hi Jono, sorry to disturb you. It's Miles from the police station. Charlie thought you might help. D'you know much about dogs?"

"Not a great deal. Four legs, bark, big teeth. Why, what's up?"

"Oh, it's Bruno, my German shepherd. He's behaving odd, seems to be panting more than usual and he's acting all... distressed."

"Where are you?"

"I'm over at the station. D'you want me to bring him to your donga?"

"No, it's OK, I'll come to you. Be there in a minute or two."

I threw the dishes in the sink and walked over to the Troopie. The sun had long since disappeared and now the mozzies were out in force. I cursed as one got me on the neck before I jumped in the cab and drove off.

Miles was waiting for me in the police station's foyer, holding the door open. "Thanks for coming, Jono. I know this is a bit left field, but you're the nearest thing we have to a vet, other than the doctors, and I didn't want to disturb them."

"No worries Miles, so where's Bruno?"

"Through here."

He showed me into an adjacent room where an enormous black German shepherd was pacing up and down. As soon as I entered, he froze and glared at me. Then his hackles raised, and he gave a menacing growl.

"Bruno, no. Down!"

He lay on the floor, complying with his master's order, but still kept his eyes fixed on me, watching my every move.

I returned the favour by scrutinising my new patient. “Well, I’m no expert, Miles, but he seems to be breathing too fast. When did this come on?”

“About half an hour ago. I’d taken him out for a walk and on the way over the playing field he picked up a stick, so I thought I’d give him a run. After a couple of throws he gave out a yelp, but returned with the stick and seemed fine, so I carried on. A bit later he slowed down, and I noticed his breathing had changed.”

He shrugged. “At first, y’know, I just thought he was rooted, so I brought him here. But... Well... he never growls at anyone like that. He’s trained not to, except on command. It’s like he’s regressed to a wild state.”

“Did you find any injuries on him?”

“No. I gave him a quick check, but with his long hair it’s difficult.”

I noticed the way the dog was glaring at me. “Have you got a muzzle for him? My patients don’t usually bite when I assess them. Well, not the sober ones, anyway.”

“Sure, I’ll be back in a second.”

Before I could reply, Miles had left, and I was alone in the room with the injured wolf-like dog. I turned to the animal and as I did, he raised himself to his feet and growled again. I tried to sound more confident than I felt and repeated Miles’ command. “Bruno, no. Down!”

Bruno ignored me, as if I was a bandicoot telling him to go eat a rabbit. Never taking my eyes off his, I used my peripheral vision to scan my surroundings, but I was in nothing more than an interview room. Even the table and chairs were bolted to the floor. Why did I let the guy with the pepper spray, taser and gun leave the room?

Bruno started moving along the wall towards me, his snout creased and lips curled back to reveal an intimidating array of teeth. Matching his determined steps, I began retreating in the opposite direction, keeping the table between us. The sparse nature of the room made me feel like I was in a lab experiment. Perhaps if I survived, I'd be rewarded with a piece of cheese. Then the thought struck me that Miles may be in another room pissing himself laughing, but what was I to do? Go pat the doggy to show how brave I was? There was no fear of that.

Suddenly the door opened and Miles walked through holding a muzzle. "Knew I had one of these somewhere, just had to find it. So, are you two getting acquainted?"

I looked at him with grateful relief and back at Bruno, who was now lying down on the floor, wagging his tail as if nothing had happened.

"What's wrong, Jono? You look like you've seen a ghost."

"I think I just met Bruno's undomesticated alter ego. If you want me to go anywhere near him, I need that muzzle on and you holding his head."

Miles looked confused. "Er… OK, Jono, whatever you say. Give me a second, I'll get this on and hold him down."

Miles attached the muzzle and sat on the floor with Bruno's head in his lap, stroking his back and whispering soothing words. "See, nothing to worry about, he's a big puppy dog, really."

"Yer, right. I think that's what they said about Cujo before he started ripping everyone to pieces."

"Cu-what?"

"Never mind. Let me have a look at him."

A few steps towards my patient were greeted by a low grumble in his chest, but I persevered. If Bruno attacked, at least there was now a gun in the room. Perhaps Miles wouldn't be able to shoot his own dog, but I sure as hell could.

I knelt down next to Bruno and started running my fingers around his body, and at one point the growl turned into a whimper. I took my hand away to find blood on my finger tips. "That doesn't look good. Can you try to stop him growling while I listen to his breathing?"

I used my stethoscope to listen to both sides of his chest, then looked straight at Miles. "You know how you didn't want to disturb the doctors? Well, we're going to have to. I think that stick jammed into his chest and punctured a lung, and what's more, it might be tensioning."

"What the hell does that mean?"

"Air is leaking into his chest and the pressure is starting to crush both his heart and the good lung. If he doesn't get it fixed soon, he'll die."

"Shit, really?"

"Hey, I'm no vet, but if we get him to the hospital, we can call one up and see what they suggest."

"OK. I guess we need to go now?"

"Yes. And he shouldn't be walking anywhere. If you carry him to the Troopie, you can lay him on the stretcher and keep him there while I drive. Let's go."

As Miles scooped up Bruno in his arms, I pulled out my phone and called the hospital. "Hi, is that Rob?"

"G'day Jono, what you got for me?"

"Bit of an unusual one tonight. How's your canine anatomy?"

"I can draw a good picture of Snoopy."

"Gonna need more than that mate. I'm bringing in Bruno the police dog with a suspected penetrating chest wound and associated pneumothorax. It might be tensioning, but I don't know what's normal obs for a dog, or where to stick the needle. What I do know is he's got a silent chest on his left side and I think he's tachycardic and hyperventilating."

"I'll call the vet in Isa. How long will you be?"

"About two minutes."

"Shit, you better get off the phone then."

I hung up and helped Miles into the back of the ambulance and drove the short distance to the hospital. Once there, I grabbed a pnuemocath set and razor from my bag, while Miles pulled the stretcher out. As we wheeled Bruno in through the A&E entrance, I noticed he was far less concerned about my presence. The double doors swung open to the sight of Gloria standing in the middle of the corridor with her hands on her hips, looking like a human roadblock.

"I don't care if it's a police dog, you're not putting it on one of my beds."

"Don't worry, Gloria, we should be able to work with him on my stretcher, it'll be a better height, anyway." The doctor walked in behind her with a phone to his ear. "Rob, where do I need to put the needle, he's going downhill fast."

"The vet says it needs to be inserted in the seventh to ninth intercostal space. She says to find the xiphoid cartilage, then move your finger up round the chest towards the spine. That rib space is the eighth and you're good to go anywhere along there."

I did as instructed and shaved a big patch of hair away with the razor. "Gloria, can you get an alcohol swab, while I prep my kit. As you're on the phone Rob, d'you mind holding Bruno down while Miles holds his head?"

"Sure."

I attached a syringe filled with saline to the large pnuemocath needle and again checked the landmarks the vet gave. "Is there anything else I need to know before jabbing him?"

"No, she's described all the same issues as with human patients, just don't delay and don't go too deep."

"Thanks."

With that, I eased the needle into Bruno's chest while pulling back on the syringe. The animal was so far gone he hardly flinched. After a few seconds I saw a stream of bubbles in the syringe, so I held the needle in place and advanced the cannula sheath into the pleural space. That done, I pulled out the needle to the hiss of escaping air.

"That should make him feel better."

In response, Bruno started whimpering and gave a wag of his tail. Even Gloria laughed and I could see Miles welling up. "Good boy, you'll be fine."

"Right, I need you all to keep a hold of him a while longer so I can get all this secured and a valve fitted."

"OK."

Once done, I had another listen to his chest. "Good equal bilateral air entry, Rob. What's the vet wanting us to do now?"

He spoke to the phone. "Got a pneumocath placed, and he's recovering. Uh-huh, yes. About a twelve gauge. That big, is it? Oh, so no need for a chest drain, right..."

The conversation continued while the rest of us watched as Bruno made a miraculous recovery. Miles grinned as he rubbed his dog's head between the ears.

Rob put his phone down. "OK, we've got to get a line in him, antibiotics on board and a little sedation to stop him ripping everything out. Then I'll check the initial wound and deal with what we find. The vet said she'll come over tomorrow on a charter flight and see how he's doing."

After Rob had sedated Bruno, Miles nipped home to fetch a wire-mesh crate and some bedding, which he set up in the waiting room. It was the closest point to the A&E that Gloria would allow. We transferred Bruno from the stretcher and hooked up a small portable medpack to monitor his condition. I was about to walk away when Miles grabbed my arm.

"Thanks, Jono. I know he's my work dog, but he means the world to me. I owe you one."

"Not a problem, Miles. His recovery's in your hands now. I'm sure you'll look after him."

"Don't you worry about that, I'll be sleeping here tonight. I'll stay with him until the vet gets here. Gotta watch out for my partner."

I pushed the stretcher back through A&E and spotted Rob. "Hey Doc, now your conference is out of the way, when's the big fishing tournament happening?"

"Meant to tell you about that, can we make it next week? I've got a paying customer."

"Wow, wonders never cease. Just as long as you're not piking out. You'll have to pay a forfeit if you do."

"What? And put up with your constant ragging? No thanks."

I started cleaning the stretcher with a disinfectant wipe. "Where you off to?"

"Oh, Pam on Sweers called. One of her guests fancies having a shot at some marlin fishing. I'm off tomorrow."

"Ha! I probably set that up for you. I've just had a few days there myself. The fishing was great…"

The ringing of my work phone interrupted our conversation. "'Scuse, Rob. Y'ello?

"Comms here. Got a call from a boat that says they've seen what looks like a ute rolled over on the beach. It's at Yuwah Point, the headland opposite Sydney Island. Are you able to go check it out?"

"Can't the caller get a better view?"

"They say they're restricted by their draught, whatever that means."

"It means the water's too shallow for their boat to approach."

"Oh, OK."

"Anyway, mark me as responding, I'm on my way."

I disconnected the phone. "Sorry Rob, gotta run. Sounds like a load of rubbish, but you'll be the first one I call if there's anything in it. I won't disturb Miles, he's got Bruno to look after."

"Well, only disturb me if it's life-threatening. I was hoping for an easy night tonight, I've got to get out early on the water tomorrow."

It took me over forty minutes to drive on the unlit dirt roads all the way to the headland. When the track ended at the coast, I could taste the dust in my mouth. I let the Troopie crawl over the dune of soft sand before the high water mark, then looked either direction along the shore. Other than the idling engine, the only sounds were the waves breaking and the ever-present chirp of cicadas. My headlights caught the white foam tips as they folded onto themselves in their endless death march to the beach. Looking through each side window, I could make out a dark shape off to my left, so I turned the Troopie in that direction and used my beams to light up the scene.

There, about a hundred metres away, was a beat up old Land Cruiser, parked on all four wheels, pointing out to sea. How would a boat have seen that from offshore and why would they think it rolled? My Spidey senses started jangling, but I depressed the accelerator and drove over to the car. A man who had been crouching down by the side of the ute stood up and walked towards me, waving his arms. As I stopped alongside him, he spoke through my open window. "It's me mate, he's got chest pain."

"Chest pain? I had this as a vehicle rollover."

"Don't know 'bout that. It's Rollo who's in trouble."

I had an inkling how the call had become confused. This guy reminded me of an artist's impression I'd seen of a Neanderthal. Crooked, yellowing teeth protruded from a mouth that looked like a torn pocket. He had a three-day growth of stubble and a high tatt-to-tooth ratio. Then I had another thought. "Didn't you report this from a boat?"

"What? Oh, I used a ship-to-shore call from the boat's radio, then came over in me tinnie."

He waved his hand in a direction past the vehicle where there was a shape of a small boat hauled up on the sand. My Spidey senses were still nagging, but his explanation seemed plausible. "OK, where is he?"

"Over there by the ute."

He pointed to what I thought was a bag of clothes propped against one wheel. "Right, I'll come check him out."

I climbed out of the cab and trudged across the wet sand to the ute. As I approached, I could see the figure of a man sitting with his arms wrapped around his legs, which were folded up against his chest. He was wearing an old cap, and his face was pressed against his knees.

I squatted down to one side of him, so he was still lit by my headlights. "Hi, my name's Jon, what's the problem? Rollo, isn't it?"

He spoke in almost a whisper without lifting his head. "Oh, Jono, I think you know who I am."

The quiet voice sparked a vague recollection and my heart froze in my chest. It couldn't be, could it? Was this the madman I'd been hunting for so many months? Had Boardie turned the tables on me yet again? Was I that easy to lure into a trap for him to exact his revenge? How stupid could I be?

The deep shadows cast by the light from the Troopie meant

the figure had taken on the quality of a satanic caricature and I felt like once more reality was merging with my dreams. But when he looked up, I recognised his weather-worn face.

"Oz? What the fuck's going on?"

It was then I felt the cold touch of gunmetal on the back of my neck and the unmistakable click of a hammer being cocked. "Don't move a muscle, Ambulance Man. We need you to come with us."

15

BLAM

I've been in plenty of stressful situations. After all, it's part of the job I do. But I always try to retain some element of control, a position within the sphere of influence. However, having a half-wit bogan jam a pistol into the base of my skull was a whole new experience. The chill of the metal seemed to permeate my skin, freezing every sinew like an injection of liquid nitrogen.

There was a flicker of a smile on Oz's face. "Hold your hands out wide and don't touch a thing on your body."

I did as he said. "What's this about, Oz? You run out of pig meat for your traps?"

The man behind me spoke. "Shut the fuck up, wise guy."

Oz reached towards me and unclipped my utility belt, letting it fall onto the ground. "Where's your personal phone?"

I nodded to my chest. "Left pocket."

He lifted it out and checked the screen. "Right. Put your hands on your head and stand up slow."

As I did, he pushed himself up using the ute as support,

his eyes never leaving mine. I thought I'd test to see what the dynamic was between these two. "C'mon Oz, I'll do what you want. Any chance you can get Monkey Boy here to ease up with the gun?"

Before he answered, the touch of metal left my neck, then a split second later pain erupted in the right side of my lower back. I dropped to my knees, unable to breathe, and fell forward, head down, fighting the urge to vomit. The cool of the wet sand on my forehead provided some relief.

As the initial shock subsided, a voice spoke in my ear, so close I could smell his stale breath. "I said, shut the fuck up. Any more crap from you and I'll punch your other kidney, then you'll be pissing blood for weeks."

"Go easy on him, Luke. We need him functioning."

"Just keepin' him in line."

"So, Jono, as you've found out the hard way, my mate here won't put up with your shit. I suggest from now on you think before you open your mouth. Now get up and start walkin' to your ambulance."

I felt the touch of metal press into my neck again and I somehow got to my feet. The ache in my flank was easing, but my mind was still spinning. What the hell did they want? Why threaten me at gunpoint? Through all the confusion, one fact stood out with arse-clenching clarity: neither of them had bothered to conceal their identity.

"Hands back on your head. Now walk."

We all moved over to the Troopie until Oz motioned for me to stop. Reaching into the cab, he pulled out a pair of vinyl gloves and slipped them on before removing the work's phone from my belt. "OK, I want you to call in, reporting this as just a mistake. The only thing you've found is some driftwood on the beach. No code words, no warnings, no bullshit. Be good and you'll walk away from this, but fuck with me and I'll use your dismembered body for croc bait."

I doubted they had any intention of letting me walk, but time might provide me with an escape plan. With Monkey Boy standing out of sight behind me, they had the angles covered, and I was pretty sure Comms wouldn't pick up on any code words. Not until it was too late. But it may be worth a try.

I nodded to him and he handed me the phone, while the gun once again dug into my neck. "Do it."

I pressed the speed dial and waited to be connected. After a few rings, a voice came on the line. "Comms here, what's the story, Mornington?"

"Hi, I'm out at the location you gave and there's nothing in this. I've searched the beach all along the headland. The only thing I found was some bleached driftwood and a couple of washed-up old tyres. I guess that's what they saw. If it's OK with you, I'll start the long return back to station."

"Hold on."

There was an extended pause, and I fantasised that someone on the other end was astute enough to pick up my LR or 'law required' reference buried in my transmission. But who was I kidding, they would just be consulting with a supervisor.

"Right, thanks for taking a look. You're clear to return."

"Cheers."

Oz plucked the mobile from my hand and disconnected the call. "See. That wasn't too difficult, was it? Now get your stuff together, we need you to check over some friends of ours."

"Friends? How many, and what's wrong with them?"

Monkey Boy spoke from behind. "If we knew what was wrong with 'em, we wouldn't need you, would we? Smart-arse."

"Well, Luke, if I'm so important could you get your fucking

gun out of my neck. I'm no use to you with a bullet through my spine."

There was a pause, then Oz nodded and after a parting jab, the gun was gone. I went to the back of the Troopie and under the watchful gaze of the other two, I pulled out the response kit, oxygen bag, and monitor.

"Can I have my belt?"

Oz held it up in the light. "Well, the phone and multitool stay here. What else d'you want?"

"My stethoscope and pen torch?"

"OK."

He took them out of their pouch and threw the rest into the cab of the Troopie, along with my personal phone. He flicked the headlights on and off three times before pulling the keys out of the ignition. The darkness was total, and I felt like a stubbie when the fridge door closed. Then Oz switched on a small flashlight.

"Right, let's go. You first, Jono."

I lugged all my kit across the sand and dumped it into the tinnie, before we all dragged the boat down to the sea. We were soon motoring away from the beach, but by then my eyes had grown accustomed to the dark. Far from being pitch black, millions of stars peppered the night's sky like a pointillist painting.

Oz was at the stern guiding the outboard, while Monkey Boy Luke was sitting on the bow facing me, pointing his gun at my midriff. I turned to look back at the island. It was now a dull shape in the distance, but our propeller was disturbing the phytoplankton in the water, leaving an eerie glow in our wake. It was a night full of natural magic and I might have enjoyed myself, if I wasn't so shit-scared.

Luke misread my glances. "Don't bother thinkin' it, Ambulance Man. You'd never make the swim. If the sharks don't get you, the crocs would. My money'd be on the crocs."

He laughed at his own humour and even in the low light I could see his crooked teeth. As I stared back at him, a dark shape loomed up in front of us, which soon took on the form of a trawler with all her lights extinguished. My immediate thought was drug smuggling. It would explain my kidnapping, but how many crew members would they need?

Luke threw the painter to another man and motioned with his gun for me to climb aboard. I handed the deck-hand my two bags and the monitor, then climbed onto the back deck. I looked around, straining my eyes in the dark, while the other three secured the tinnie. Pervading the usual smells of diesel, dead fish and oil was the pungent aroma of fresh cigars. An orange disc of light flared in the shadows, and I could hear the slight crackle as the rolled leaves smouldered from the air sucked through them.

A voice that suggested decades of smoke and alcohol abuse growled out from the gloom. "Leave your stuff there an' follow me."

I did as he ordered and we climbed the stairs to the bridge. Once inside, he flipped on a light and I finally saw the boss of the operation. He bore a striking resemblance to Luke, about ten years older, but looking smarter and meaner. He glared at me as if I were to blame for whatever crisis had occurred on his ship.

"You're here to check my passengers. There's somethin' wrong with 'em and I need you to fix 'em."

"I can't promise that."

"Well, you better hope you can as it's the only fuckin' way you're getting off here alive."

I stared into his cold eyes and he took another pull on his

cigar. Whatever happened, my longevity was not a concern for this man. "What symptoms do they have?"

He blew out some smoke before speaking. "It all started with their skin itching, then a few of them lost the feelings in their legs. Now, well, take a look."

He opened a cabinet and turned on a TV screen that showed four grainy images from inside what seemed to be a small dormitory. Most of the people were writhing around in their bunks, but the sound feed was the most disturbing. A cacophony of groans and weeping came from the speakers, punctuated by the odd scream.

I stared at the video. "How many are there?"

"Twenty."

"Christ. When did it start?"

"About two hours ago."

"Has anyone else been affected, other than those in your hold?"

His cigar tip glowed and when he exhaled, the smoke billowed around his face. "No and they're not in the hold."

I was confused. "So where are they? Can I go see them?"

"They're in a container we've been towing behind us."

"A container? Towing? D'you mean underwater?"

"Yes."

"How deep?"

"Most of the time, 'bout nine metres."

"And let me guess, the symptoms came on when you raised them to the surface."

"Yes."

"Well, that's your problem. I'd have to check them over, but it sounds like Caisson disease, y'know, decompression sickness. They're all bent."

He shook his head. "No fuckin' way, already thought of that. It's not possible; the tables only start at ten metres, it's why I towed them at nine. They haven't been deep enough to get the bends."

"How long have you been towing them?"

"About a week."

"A week! Holy shit! Just because recreational dive tables don't have figures for less than ten metres, doesn't mean the pressure won't affect them. They've been breathing hyperbaric air for seven days. Those tables were designed for a few hours scuba diving at the most. Their tissues would be super-saturated with nitrogen. Bring them to the surface too quick and bubbles will form. That's what's causing their symptoms."

He folded his arms and chewed on his cigar. "So what you gonna do about it?"

"Me? They need a recompression chamber and a diving doctor, not a paramedic."

"Well, all we've got is you. And as you've probably guessed, we can't deliver these fuckers to the nearest hospital, so you better come up with some sort of plan, otherwise you'll be joining them all at the bottom of the Gulf."

I leant back on a map table and considered my options as Oz walked onto the bridge. "So, does he know what's wrong with 'em?"

"Reckons they've got the bends."

Oz looked at me. "Thought that wasn't possible? Anyways, you're a paramedic from Brisbane. How d'you know what the bends looks like?"

"And you're a fucked-up old fisherman. What d'you know about people smuggling?"

He stepped towards me with a clenched fist, but the skipper stopped his advance. "Oz has a point. How the fuck d'you know so much about it?"

I shrugged. "Grew up in Townsville. I was always on boats and did a lot of diving." I threw my hands open wide. "Look, it fits with the timescale and the variety of symptoms. Skin bends, or 'The Creeps', comes on first. That's the itchy feeling. It doesn't usually happen with scuba, but they often come on from being in hyperbaric chambers… Hold on. How deep can you take that container?"

"It's good for at least forty metres."

"Well, there's your answer. Take them down to twenty and the nitrogen bubbles will go back into solution. Then raise them over a much longer time frame to give them a chance to off-gas."

"How long?"

I gave another shrug. "I don't know, twelve hours?"

The skipper looked at his watch and grimaced. "We've only got eight hours of darkness for the plane to come in and take them out."

I shook my head. "Whoa, hold on, they can't fly! The reduced pressure at altitude will bring on the bends again."

"Well, they ain't fuckin' stayin' in that container. How long d'they need before they can fly?"

"Not a clue. I'm pretty sure it's twelve hours surface time after a single dive, but that's when you haven't suffered a bend."

"Fuck."

He chewed hard on his cigar and glanced at Oz, who shrugged. "We could get the plane to come tomorrow, say midnight."

The skipper nodded. "If I took 'em down to twenty, I could raise 'em to a few metres by sunrise. They could sit there under the boat for the daylight hours, so no one can see 'em. Then I'll bring 'em to the surface after dark. D'you reckon that'd be fuckin' slow enough, Ambulance Man?"

"Probably, but it doesn't deal with the plane issue."

The skipper glared at me, but Oz broke the tension. "Hey,

we're not filing any flight plan here. If the pilot stays away from any settlements, he could fly close to the ground all the way to the Kombi vans."

Oz received a reproachful glance from the skipper and my feelings of impending doom sank deeper than the seabed. I now knew far too much about their operation to stand any chance of release. If I was to survive this ordeal, it would have to be under my own steam.

The skipper seemed to relax a little and took a slow draw on his cigar while he looked me up and down. "So, what d'you need to take with you?"

"Let me guess, I'm going in the container?"

He smiled at Oz. "You said he was smart fucker."

He then turned back to me. "Someone's gotta look after 'em, and it sure as fuck ain't gonna be me. So, I'll ask you again, what d'you need to take with you?"

I thought for a moment. "A shitload of oxygen."

"Oxygen? Why?"

"Partial pressures… Don't worry, all you need to know is that they'll lose nitrogen faster. I've only got one small cylinder with me and another in the Troopie, along with two large ones. For twenty people I'll need far more, so someone'll have to get as much as they can from the station."

"No fuckin' way. Anything else?"

"That wasn't an optional extra. Even if they were being treated in a hyperbaric centre, they'd be on oxygen. It's the primary treatment for the bends. If you want them to have any chance of flying out tomorrow night, you need to get me as much of the stuff as possible."

He chewed on his cigar again. "Fuck, this just keeps getting better. Oz, you able to sort this?"

The fisherman rubbed his chin. "Well, his ambulance needs returning to the station pretty soon coz of that transponder thing. So I'll get Luke to follow me in my ute and bring back the oxygen. It's still going to take a while with that other stuff I've got to do."

"How long?"

He shrugged. "Two hours, at least."

"Shit, is there anything we can do for them in the meantime?"

Oz and the skipper looked at me.

"What depth are they at now?"

"Just below the surface."

"You could drop them to ten metres, it should ease their symptoms. But you'll have to bring them back up to get me and the oxygen in. I guess it'd be worth trying, and at the least it'll confirm the cause."

"Right. Oz, go now, but take Bruce with you. D'you need any stuff from your bags, Ambulance Man, 'cos they're going with him."

"My name's Jon."

"D'you think I give a flying fuck what you're called?"

I shrugged. "Don't know, but you do seem to care a lot about your passengers. I thought people smugglers didn't give two shits about their cargoes."

"They're on a guaranteed delivery. You, on the other hand, are expendable. So, keep your fuckin' thoughts to yourself, Ambulance Man."

Twisting my cable-tied wrists over, I looked at my watch. Two and half hours… they were late. I clenched my arse cheeks to ease the pain from sitting on the hard wooden floor of the bridge. Luke was leaning against a wall next to the door, training his gun in my general direction. I'd thought of rushing him, but the skipper had positioned us well. It would take far too long for me to close the distance, plus the map table was in the way.

Dropping the container down to ten metres had at least stopped the groaning from the TV speakers, and most of my patients seemed to have opted for a restless sleep. Except one woman wearing a black hijab. She paced the limited space like a caged lion and kept staring up at the cameras. She looked less than impressed at her plight.

After they'd been down for an hour, I'd asked the skipper to raise them in preparation for my internment, and now I could see some were starting to scratch. When they reached sea level, the skipper left Luke in charge and went to secure the container alongside the trawler.

I thought I'd take the opportunity to wind up the simpleton. "D'you think Oz has done a runner?"

"Shut the fuck up."

"He should be back by now. Perhaps he's reported you to the cops. Maybe he'll get a reward."

"I said…"

"I heard you, Luke, but what're you going to do? You need me to treat those poor bastards in that box and after they're gone, you'll kill me. So tell me, why should I shut the fuck up?"

"Your death can be quick, or I can make it very slow."

"No offence, Luke, but did you get that from a movie? I don't reckon you've seen a dead body, let alone murdered someone. I'm surprised your brother trusted you with that gun. Have you checked he left any rounds in it?"

He cocked the hammer and pointed the weapon at my head. "Course he fuckin' did, now stop talkin' or I'll prove it's loaded."

His nostrils were flaring and eyes darting, so I thought I'd better ease off. I turned my gaze to the TV screen where the woman was once again scratching her arms. They were getting more symptomatic. If Oz didn't get back soon, the joint pains would return and so would the groaning. Out of the corner of my eye, I caught sight of Luke pointing the gun towards himself and looking into the barrel. Jesus, was he really that stupid?

BLAM!

The howl of the weapon discharging echoed around the bridge. My mouth fell open, and I stared at Luke as he stared at me. A perfect hole had appeared right in the centre of his forehead and a trickle of blood traced a path down his nose. The next second the door flew open and the skipper burst in. "What the f..."

Luke's upper body relaxed against the wall and his head rested on the brain matter that was sprayed up to the ceiling behind him. His arms dropped to his side, and the gun made a metallic thud as it fell from his hand. Then his knees buckled, and he slid into a crumpled heap on the floor.

I sat absolutely still, not daring to breathe. I braced myself for the inevitable outrage about to follow, and I knew the focus would be on me. The skipper stared at his brother's body as the acrid odour of gunpowder mixed with the sickly sweet smell of blood. My ears were ringing from the gunshot, but over the silence of the room I heard an approaching outboard.

The skipper sighed and shook his head. "Oh for Christ's sake Luke, you just had a few more minutes not to fuck up."

To my amazement, he retrieved the gun from the floor and waved it at me. "Get up. It's time for you to go to work."

Waves lapped around the sides of what looked like a dark-grey shipping container. However, it was floating about a metre out of the water, supported by a complicated framework, which I presumed allowed them to control its depth. Integrated into the chassis were two large tubes resembling mini-submarines, each with their own prop, and the front of the frame was shaped to provide streamlining.

As I came down the stairs, Bruce jumped onto the back deck and secured the painter. The skipper called from behind me. "Took your fuckin' time, what was the holdup?"

Bruce shrugged. "There were only two large cylinders at the ambulance station, so Oz thought the ones at the hospital were less likely to be missed. But we had to be quiet and so loadin' them was fuckin' slow."

Oz swung himself over the gunwale. "Got eight of the big bastards and a couple of small uns. Also sorted out that other issue. The whole thing took more time than expected."

"Yes, well there's been a..." The skipper sighed. "Luke fuckin' shot himself while I was sorting the rig out."

"Fuck, is he OK?"

"No, Bruce, he's not. He's fuckin' dead, so now we've got one less pair of hands to sort out this fuckin' mess."

The skipper chewed on the butt of his cigar as a chilling silence engulfed the deck. Bruce was the first to respond. "Dead? How?"

"Look, we haven't time for this. My fuckwit brother just blew his own fuckin' head off when he was watchin' this cunt. Now can we get a fuckin' move on?"

There was another pause while everyone stared at the skipper, then Oz headed back to the tinnie. "C'mere Bruce, I'll hand you the cylinders. Stack them up over there."

As they worked, the skipper turned to me and used a knife to cut my cable tie. "Don't think of doing anything smart while you're down there, Ambulance Man. I've got a kill switch in the bridge. You fuck with me and the container'll fill with water and sink to the bottom. Y'understand?"

I nodded. I'd seen many responses to the death of loved ones, some more overt than others. But his reaction to Luke's premature demise showed he didn't give a damn about anyone other than himself.

He then barked out another order. "Bruce, when you've got the cylinders on board, jump on the container and open it up."

Without a murmur, Bruce did as he was told.

The skipper looked at me. "Once he opens the hatch, climb down and we'll pass you the oxygen."

"Right."

Bruce jumped from the deck onto the roof of the container and walked over to a point about a third of the way along. He released a concealed panel, sliding it aside to reveal a circular stainless steel wheel atop a watertight hatch. After a slight struggle, he spun the handle, and the door swung inwards on its hinges. He wrinkled his nose and wafted a hand in front of his face. "Jesus, it stinks down there."

The skipper nodded to me. "Over you go, Ambulance Man."

I picked up the carrier bag of items they'd let me take from my kit and clambered onto the container with far less grace than Bruce had managed. With a couple of slipping steps on the wet metal, I was soon looking through the opening, down into a dim interior that emanated a strong body odour. I sighed and lowered myself to the ladder and climbed down into a living hell.

As soon as my feet reached the floor, my neck was pinned in a headlock and I was shoved against the rungs, the impact forcing out my breath. I attempted to move, but the arm tightened its grip. Then a female voice spoke in my ear. "Who're you?"

I tried to respond, but my compressed larynx could only manage a muffled grunt. She eased her hold so I could speak. "Jon. My name's Jon. I'm a paramedic here to help you."

"This wasn't the plan."

"Neither was you guys getting the bends."

"The bends? They said that wasn't possible."

"They were wrong."

There was a pause and for the second time in a matter of hours I could feel someone's breath on my ear. Then the arm was gone and I could breathe again. I turned to see my assailant, who had retreated as far as the cramped conditions allowed. She seemed ready to lash out. A cornered animal, but a beautiful one at that. Her vivid green eyes were enough to capture the soul of even the most chaste man, but she looked as dangerous as a mythical siren. Her black hijab gave her a ninja-like appearance, with her stance and posture revealing combat training, and the position of her hand suggesting a concealed weapon.

I dropped the bag and raised my open hands, showing her my palms. "I'm unarmed. You have nothing to fear from me."

Her position didn't change, apart from her eyes that watched my every move. Then the skipper yelled down. "They all got their hoods on?"

I looked over to the bunks where a black hood covered each occupant's head. The woman called up. "Yes."

"Right, Ambulance Man, here come your cylinders."

I pointed to the opening, still not wanting to make any undue moves. "I need oxygen to treat you all. They're going to pass down some cylinders."

She nodded her agreement, and I reached up to take the first gas bottle. After they were all loaded, a hand grabbed the hatch, swinging it up with a slam. Then there was a spinning sound as the wheel tightened. A few minutes later, an intercom crackled into life. "Brace yourself, Ambulance Man, you're all going down."

I held onto the ladder. "Everyone listen up! Take your hoods off and get ready to clear your ears. We're descending to twenty metres. My name's Jon and I'm here to help you. The pain and itching you've been suffering have been due to the bends caused by nitrogen bubbles."

I grabbed my nose and blew to equalise my ears. "The only way I can treat you is to put you back under pressure, then slowly return you to the surface. This'll give your bodies enough time to release the nitrogen. I'm going to assist the process by flushing the room with oxygen."

While I was blowing on my nose again, the woman spoke. "Most of them can't speak much English."

"Right. Of course. Can you translate?"

She began calling out in a language I didn't recognise, while I reflected on my situation. Twenty bent patients who hardly speak English, a handful of cannulas, a few drugs and not even one monitor to share around. The scenario kept getting better.

The intercom interrupted my thoughts. "That's twenty."

I gave my ears a last tweak, then started opening the valves on the big cylinders. The lower the percentage of nitrogen in the inhaled air, the more of the gas would be released with each breath. It would be preferable if every patient was breathing neat oxygen through a mask, but only the two small cylinders had built-in regulators, so this was my best option. The small ones might come in handy if any of my patients needed special attention.

I walked around the room, tapping each person on the shoulder and giving them a thumbs up. A few shook their heads, but most returned the signal, apart from a man in one of the bottom bunks. He was unconscious.

I dragged him out onto the floor to assess him. He still had a pulse and was breathing, but my knuckles pressing hard on his sternum only elicited a disinterested groan.

"How long's he been like this?"

The woman shrugged. "About three days."

"What?"

"I had to sedate him."

"Why?"

"His ears. A few days ago we had to go deep, and he went crazy."

"What did you use to sedate him?"

She shook her head. "I don't know. They gave me unlabelled syringes to use in an emergency."

"Great. When did you give the last one?"

"About an hour ago. The drug seems to work for six, then he starts screaming again."

"Did he have any problems before the deep dive?"

She shrugged, but a man with a bushy moustache waved at me from a bunk. "I answer that, yes?"

"Please. Go on."

"His name Nasim. His ears having pains ever since underwater. But he good, give us all English lesson. I worry about him, no. He took too much white pills."

"White pills?"

"They give us bottle for anxious, but he eat lots. I give him some of my own tablets, decon... Deconjugant with opiate?"

"Decongestant?"

"Yes, yes. Decongestant. Sorry, my English crap."

"It's a hell of a lot better than any other language I can speak. How long after you gave him your tablets did he go crazy?"

He shrugged. “Six… seven hour?”

“OK, thanks for that.”

I turned to the woman, who appeared to have relaxed a little. “When you said he went crazy, what did he do exactly?”

Her face was impassive. “He held his head and started screaming. Dropped to his knees, then vomited. Afterwards, he didn’t appear to hear anything, and began crawling around on the floor. Then he staggered to his feet and pulled the emergency alarm. I had to subdue him.”

“I thought she kill him.”

Another man joined in. “Me too, he look dead.”

“Well, evidently he isn’t, but he’s probably got a severe barotrauma to one or both of his ears.”

The woman furrowed her brow and I realised I was using medical terms with non-clinicians.

“Sorry, his ears are damaged by the pressure changes. They’re usually associated with diving accidents, or sometimes explosions. You guys should be fine by the time we reach the surface, but there’s no doubt he’ll need a hospital.”

She looked alarmed. “Hospital? Why?”

“He’s probably ruptured his inner ear.”

“So? Won’t his hearing get better?”

“Hearing’s not the only thing the inner ear does, it also provides you with the sense of balance. He may require surgery to repair the damage, but even if he doesn’t, he won’t be able to stand for quite some time without vomiting.”

16

STRANDLINE

"G'day Charlie, it's Albert."

"Yer, I know. Your name comes up on my phone, eh. What's up?"

"Have you seen Jono? He hasn't shown up for our meeting and he's not in his donga."

"Thought your meetings were on Thursday, eh?"

"Yes, well, I was off sick yesterday and I had to postpone, but we were supposed to meet today. Plus the fact, he's not answering his, or the work's phone. Just wondered if you'd seen him?"

"No, but I'm not up to much, I'll have a look around, eh. Leave it with me Albert, I'll get back to you."

"Thanks."

Charlie hung up and pocketed the device. Surely Jono wouldn't be so stupid as to get pissed on a workday? Guess there was always a first time. He sighed and pushed the chair out from behind him. He knew how hard it could be to fight those personal battles, and it was something he didn't want to dwell on too much. But Jono had plenty of reasons to be screwed up; he just needed some help to get through things.

He swept up his hat off its peg as he left the house and pulled the brim down on his forehead. Swinging himself into the cab of his ute, he drove away with a slight spin of the tyres.

Before leaving town, he thought he'd check the jetty. Never know, Jono might've taken his advice and switched off his mobile. But when he arrived, he could see Jono wasn't any of the three figures sitting under the shade. Still, he thought he better find out if he'd been there.

He parked his ute and wandered out along the wooden structure, glancing down at the shoreline where he'd jumped on the croc. He smiled to himself. Punch was a good nickname. We all do stupid things, but at least that event had a happy ending.

He called out as he approached the others. "G'day fellas. Catchin' much?"

Pete nodded to him. "Ain't brought in your sailfish if that's what you're askin'.

The three men chuckled at Charlie's expense and he nodded his head. "Never gonna live that one down, eh."

"Nope, not in my lifetime."

"Eh, any of you seen Jono?"

They shook their heads, but Pete raised a finger. "Saw him here yestdee, eh."

"But not this morning?"

"No, hold on. Yestdee was barge day, eh." The old man nodded to himself. "I seen 'im the day before. When he come back in 'is boat, eh."

"So no one's seen him this mornin' then?"

They all shook their heads again.

"Thanks."

"He ain't in any trouble, is he Charlie?"

"I hope not, Thomas, I sure hope not."

It didn't take Charlie long to drive out to Gee Wee Point. The apprehension that started at the jetty had gnawed its way from his belly to his chest like some medieval rat torture. As he pulled up to the shore, the sun was almost straight overhead. Rays shimmered off the calm water of the Gulf and seared the golden sand, causing him to squint despite his sunnies. With the outside temperature pushing forty, he conducted his search from inside the air-conditioned cab, but his heart sank as he spotted the table and chair.

Driving over to the camp furniture, he jumped from his ute, hardly noticing the scorching heat of the day. Near the chair an empty bottle of Bundaberg rum lay on its side amidst the rucked-up sand. At an angle coming up the beach were what looked like croc tracks, with drag marks extending straight down to the water, which was gently lapping the shore. Something glinted among the washed up seagrass of the strandline that caught his attention. Looking closer, he recognised the shape. Not wanting to disturb the scene any more than he had to, he reached in his pocket and pulled out his mobile, pressing one of the speed dials. A few seconds later, Jono's ringtone echoed around the beachfront.

17

NYSTAGMUS

I sat on a pillow with my back against the cold metal wall. These guys had lasted two weeks in this box, but I'd had enough after only a few hours. Although I had little to do, boredom was not a concern when I had less than a day to live. Why did shit like this keep happening to me? What did I do to deserve it? Just when I found a way to sort out my life after the last butt fucking, along comes a band of cut-throats ready to rip down my pants.

I sighed and looked around. I'd located three of the four cameras and had a good idea of the fourth's whereabouts. Although it was only a modified shipping container, it must have represented a significant outlay. My best chance of survival in the short term was to stay inside the enclosure. The hatch was narrow and easy to defend, while the likelihood of the skipper dumping the whole box just to deal with me seemed an expensive option.

I'd done the rounds a few times, checking on how everyone was doing. Apart from belonging to different nationalities and speaking broken English, they all appeared to be normal people. Normal people prepared to go to extraordinary lengths to flee persecution or threats to their lives. But something had struck me about the group. None were destitute. None were uneducated. They were all professionals; an accountant, a dentist, two engineers, the list went on. And another thing: almost all were men, except for one who had come with her husband and, of course, the green-eyed woman.

On a clinical level, they were all dehydrated to varying degrees, which is a predisposing factor for the bends. But my efforts to get them to drink had failed. Apparently, consuming everyone else's processed urine was a fate worse than agonising joint pain. I would have drunk the water; it was filtered. Then again, I don't like pain.

My last thought focused my attention back to Nasim. From the limited amount of assessment I could do, he was in a bad way, not least from being sedated for three days. He felt cold and there was a pressure sore on his elbow. I had nothing to treat his wounds, so I didn't see the point of checking the rest of his body. I guessed they hadn't told his surrogate nurse to keep him warm and roll him over. Mind you, I doubt they expected anyone would need sedating for that long.

The drug was yet to wear off, but I'd taken the opportunity to cannulate him and administered some morphine, along with an anti-emetic to help with the nausea. If he had an inner-ear rupture, then recompressing him was likely to make things worse rather than better. But no one warned me how serious he was.

I looked up to find the green-eyed woman watching me, leaning against the opposite wall, arms folded. I returned her gaze, but if the eyes are the windows to the soul, hers had curtains. Either that or there was no soul behind those emerald irises.

She kept staring back, and I spoke before I had to blink.

"So, what's your rank?"

"Do you always try to read people?"

"It's part of my job."

"I thought you were a paramedic."

"I am. Prehospital medicine's an unpredictable environment; I need to know when a patient's lying or not telling the whole truth. And understanding when it's safe to approach is essential. Believe me, I've been in all sorts of situations." I looked around and shrugged. "Mind you, this is something new."

She went back to her mute stare.

"So, what's a pretty girl like you doin' in a place like this?"

Nothing. Not even the flicker of a smile, or frown.

"C'mon, how d'you end up working for a bunch of people smugglers?"

"I don't work for them."

"Riiight."

"I'm just another passenger."

"With a martial arts background?"

She let out a short laugh and shook her head.

"What, you deny it? When I came down that ladder, you had me immobilised and breathless before I knew what was happening, and you were only using one arm. That takes training."

She went to respond, but then turned and walked off to the other set of bunks, out of my line of sight. In that moment I caught a glimpse, for a fraction of a second, of the slightest facial expression. What was it? Annoyance, frustration, anger? Somehow I'd got a reaction. Despite herself. Despite her… training?

"Psst."

It was the man with the moustache. "Well done. That the most she say in two week."

"Really?"

"Most of us scared of her. She call herself Tshaarre. It mean 'knife' in Pashto."

"Great. And I'm guessing she's not a chef."

He chuckled just as my patient groaned and pushed himself up to a sitting position.

"Hello Nasim. Do you speak English?"

He still appeared groggy, and was yet to open his eyes. "Yes… Who are you?"

"Jon. I'm a paramedic here to help."

His body tensed and his lids shot up. As he attempted to focus on me, I noticed his eyes were moving in a characteristic jerky motion, known as nystagmus, or dancing eyes. One of the causes was inner-ear damage.

I tried to calm him. "Don't worry, you're still in the container and you haven't been discovered. On the other hand, I've been kidnapped, so I'm in a world of shit."

"Everything keeps jumping, what's going on?"

"It's your eyes. You've got inner-ear damage, it affects your eye movement. Tilting your head back might help, or just close your eyes."

He extended his head back and squinted at me, but then screwed his eyes closed.

"What's that noise?"

"Noise?"

He hesitated. "Can't you hear it? It's like a high-pitched bell, constant, but rising and falling in waves. I can hardly hear you."

I smiled at him. "It's called tinnitus, mate. Again, it's because the pressure changes in here damaged your ears."

He opened one wavering eye. "Can you do anything?"

"Not here, I'm afraid. I've given you pain relief and something to stop you feeling sick, but you need to see a specialist."

He sighed and closed his eyes. A tear trickled down the side of his face. "My hearing's my livelihood. I'm a translator."

"Really? What languages?"

"Pardon?"

I raised my voice. "What languages do you speak?"

"The main Afghan ones such as Pashto, Dari, Uzbek, and Turkmen, but also Urdu and other variants of Persian." He managed a wry smile. "Not to mention Balochi, Pashayi, Nuristani, Pamiri, and about ten other dialects."

"Wow. That's impressive. Hey, other than English, I know Australian, American, Canadian, Kiwi, and a bit of Scottish."

His smile became a little warmer. "Sounds like you're fluent in bullshit as well, my friend. But if I'd stuck to one language, I wouldn't be in this mess."

"How so?"

He repositioned himself against the wall. "I worked for the Australian military and most of your soldiers are pulling out of my country next month. They refused to give us assurances they'd relocate all their interpreters, so my parents decided it was safer to smuggle me out."

He shrugged. "They're wealthy, and I'm far too idealistic for my own good. I thought the coalition forces would at least stay until there was some sort of peace. But the Taliban are more patient than Western politicians."

"Too true. The pollies can't think past the next election."

He rubbed his face, giving special attention to his eyes. "It feels like my head is full to bursting and the pain is building again."

"Here, I need your left hand, there's a cannula in it. I'll give you another shot of morphine, but you should rest. If you can, try sleeping sitting up, it'll help with your ears."

He opened one eye for a moment and gave me a slight nod. "Thank you."

18

LUKEWARM

Detective Giallo swung open the door and walked into the spacious office. "Did you see the news?"

The Chief frowned at the intruder. "Haven't you heard of knocking, Detective?"

"Sorry, Chief. D'you want me to go out and knock?"

Giallo's boss rocked back in his leather executive wheelie chair, which creaked as his bulk shifted. He placed his hands behind his head revealing two large sweat patches around the armpits of his shirt. He then gave Giallo a look that would have impressed Medusa. "What is it?"

Giallo turned and closed the door before addressing his superior. "It's the ambo, Jonothan Byrne."

"Oh Christ. What's he done now?"

"Nothing, apart from go missing."

"Missing? Again?"

"They think he's been taken by a croc."

His eyebrows shot up and his jowls wobbled. "A croc?"

"Y'know, I told you. He's working up on Mornington Island, Far North Queensland. It turns out they've been trying to catch a big one up there ever since it grabbed a boy near the jetty."

He shook his head. "Fuck. What a way to go."

There was an awkward silence as he stared back at his detective, expecting some sort of response, but Giallo just stood there.

"Oh no, it's that gut instinct of yours again, isn't it?"

Giallo walked forward and sat down in front of the Chief's desk. "Well, you know how I've tracked our serial killer, Darren Boardman, to Indonesia?"

"C'mon, that's a bit of a stretch, even for you."

"Hey, it's his MO. Murders made to look like natural deaths."

"But travelling all the way to Mornington Island to snatch an ambo?"

"You can't say he's not the type to hold a grudge."

Giallo angled side-on to his boss and rested an elbow on his desk, peering into the open box of Krispy Kreme donuts. "One of those for me?"

"No. So what else d'you want?"

"Just let me go up there and check things out. It's almost exactly a year since Jono's girlfriend was murdered. I feel like there's something fishy about the whole thing."

"What, more than crocodile breath?" He laughed at his own joke.

"Not funny Chief, he might've been eaten by one."

His face returned to its usual scowl. "Thought you didn't believe it?"

"I could be wrong."

He sighed and leant forward onto his desk. "Look, I know you're still after Boardman, but I can't sanction a wild goose chase for you to investigate a cold case."

"It's not cold."

"Really?"

"OK, I'll accept lukewarm."

"Whatever. When was the last time you had a holiday, Giallo? You must have a pretty healthy leave balance. If it means so much to you, go have yourself a tropical vacation and I'll sign off on your application."

Giallo stood up and snatched a donut before making for the door. "Thanks Chief, see you in a week or so. The paperwork's already in your pigeon hole. I've got to dash, I'm booked on tomorrow's 9:00 AM flight to The Isa."

19

LANDMARK

Early in the morning, the skipper announced we'd reached two metres and other than a couple of people complaining of some mild itchy patches, none of the more severe symptoms had returned. But Nasim was a different story. Halfway through the day the morphine ran out and the pain in his head became so intense I too had to resort to sedation, though only in small doses. He'd still have to climb out of the container when it was his turn.

I looked at my watch for the hundredth time and wondered if 'The Knife' would live up to her name before or after the others had left. I'd been racking my brain for how to defend myself, how to stay alive, but so far I'd drawn a blank. Jabbing her with a syringe full of midazolam was pointless, as an intramuscular dose never worked as fast as sedatives used in the movies. She'd have plenty of time to slice, dice, and start a casserole with me before the drug took effect. And that was presuming I could get anywhere near her. She had considered the likelihood of me making some sort of attack, for at no point did she come within lunging distance. But who was I trying to fool? A few lessons of karate as a kid hardly qualified me for taking on a trained killer, if that's what she was.

I sighed and glanced at my watch again - 10:15 PM. Five minutes after I last looked. Shit. What was I going to do? Everyone must know I'm missing by now. Perhaps they've sent search parties out to the beach where I went for that call. Perhaps they've spotted the trawler and the cavalry's on its way.

What the fuck was I thinking? Why would a trawler offshore raise any suspicions? They often use the lee of the island for safe anchorage. Come to think of it, Oz mentioned needing to return the ambulance because of its transponder. That meant they must have concocted a cover story for my disappearance. If I sit and wait for the cavalry, I'll be as dead as Custer.

I jumped as the skipper's voice boomed through the container. "Put your hoods on, we'll be moving you out in groups of five."

Everyone climbed from their bunks and placed their head coverings on, like the automatic actions of the Eloi from 'The Time Machine'. That is, except for myself and my own personal Morlock, who stood near the hatch, watching my every move with her cold green eyes. Nasim also failed to heed the call, lying on the floor propped against the wall, fast asleep. I left him there. It would make sense that he exited with the last group.

As for the others, there was a slight buzz of anticipation. Not only were they being released from their underwater confinement, but this was the start of their new lives, a back-door entry into the lucky land. I bore them no animosity; it's natural to seek a safe place to live, somewhere you can settle down and perhaps raise a family. I just wanted to extend my own life past their departure.

There was a spinning sound, and the hatch dropped open with a clank, accompanied by a splash of seawater.

Bruce shouted down. "OK, send 'em up."

The woman guided an occupant over to the ladder, and he climbed out of sight. When the fifth was making his way up, she addressed the room. "That's five, the rest of you stay."

She repeated the instruction in two other languages, while a hand reached down and slammed the hatch shut and another wait began. I felt my heart thumping in my chest and my muscles tensing, but there was nothing I could do. There were still too many people obstructing the walkway to attempt anything against my attractive adversary, and she was well aware of that. I had to focus on trying to maintain my casual body language, hoping she couldn't read my mounting anxiety.

Everyone stood there in their hoods, the container swaying in the slight swell now that we were on the surface. No one said a word. In the hushed silence, I heard the buzz of the outboard motor departing with the first batch of refugees. Then nothing but the drip of a tap. The quiet of the room amplified the sound of the intermittent splash and as it dripped away, it became like an auditory Chinese water torture.

"Mind if I switch the tap off?"

Tshaarre nodded, and I moved over to the sink and tightened the faucet. And we were back to the silence. I returned to my slouched position against the wall and rubbed my face, yawning. I hadn't slept for about forty hours, but my brain was wired. Funny how imminent death can act as a stimulant.

It took over twenty minutes for the boat to return, and the tension in the container was palpable. Another five climbed out, and we were once again sealed in our metal tomb with the silence dragging on. But then a grin spread across my face and I managed to squeeze out a loud fart.

Tshaarre glared at me, while several people started giggling. I recognised Rashid's voice from under his hood. "Hope that not smell."

Before I replied, someone else let rip and the few giggles soon blossomed into full-on laughter that echoed off the metal walls. Every time the silence threatened to return, there was another bout of flatulence and the group once again fell into hysterics.

Before long my sides were aching, but I managed to say, "Guess that's one language we're all fluent in."

Tshaarre, who had remained tight-lipped throughout, cut through the laughter. "Be quiet! All of you!"

You could hear a pin drop until I dropped my guts again, and we were all laughing until the hatch swung down about ten minutes later.

"Five more, now."

They climbed the ladder, still sniggering, and the hatch clanked shut on the remaining occupants.

With only three hooded refugees and one asleep, I recognised the dynamics had changed, but I tried to continue the frivolity. It was helping to hide my unease. "And then there were six. Anyone know a song?"

Tshaarre's response was a hiss. "Sing and I'll feed you your own tongue."

"Guess that's a 'no' then."

"Silence!"

"Or what? You'll kill me? The skipper promised me a safe return if I fixed you guys."

"Did he." She said it as a statement rather than a question.

"Perhaps you should discuss it with him? I wouldn't want you getting in trouble with your boss."

"He's not my boss."

"So, who is your boss? Why would a Muslim woman with

combat training need unannounced illegal access into Australia? Got a date with destiny?"

She glared at me. "Why do Westerners always assume that everyone wearing a hijab is a terrorist?"

"I don't, but you're the one using the word. I guess, if the shoe fits."

She frowned. "If the shoe fits, what?"

"It's an expression. If the shoe fits, then wear it. Maybe your English isn't as good as you thought. Making a mistake like that might blow your cover."

She sighed. "I'm not undercover, I'm just a refugee like the rest. They gave me a discount if I controlled things down here. Now be quiet while we wait."

I adjusted my slouch against the wall and folded my arms. Could I have misread her? Was I losing my touch? My Spidey senses told me otherwise, and if I'd listened to them back on the beach, perhaps I wouldn't be here. I started humming a tune and although I was aware of her staring at me, she didn't attempt another reprimand.

After a while, the sound of the returning outboard caused me to stop. I clapped my hands and rubbed them together. "Right. Guess the rest of us climb out now. I'm famished. Those protein drinks you've got down here taste like shit."

The hatch swung open, and I gave Nasim a nudge. "C'mon sleeping beauty. You need to get up, it's time to go."

"Move away! I'll see to him."

I held up my palms. "Whatever you say, just trying to help."

As she guided the other three up the ladder, I backed off along the central corridor, giving myself some room to manoeuvre. Once the last set of feet disappeared, she turned her attention to Nasim and crouched in front of him.

This was my opportunity, this was my chance, the moment

I'd been waiting for. I grabbed the handle of one of the small oxygen cylinders, but hesitated when I saw what she was doing. The woman I thought was a hard-nosed killer was cradling Nasim's head, stroking the back of his neck, as if gently waking him.

However, what I mistook for a caress was in fact a search for the correct anatomical landmark, much as I'd done when finding where to push the needle into Bruno's chest.

But this was no life-saving intervention.

Her free hand whipped out a short black knife and plunged it into Nasim's neck, just below the skull, severing his spinal cord. His body made a brief shudder, then went limp. My split second of confusion had cost Nasim his life.

I screamed and swung the cylinder with all my might, intending to smash her head, but my cry gave her the warning she needed. She dropped to one side and held up her left arm to deflect the blow. Lucky for me, she'd underestimated my rage and not anticipated a weapon. The oxygen bottle impacted her forearm with a sickening crack and she let out a shriek of her own. I brought up the cylinder for a second strike, but as it passed my chest, there was a thud followed by a hissing sound. Wounded, but not down, she'd thrown her blade, which was now embedded in the oxygen tank.

"Fuck."

As she reached for another knife, I backed off to the other row of bunks and hid behind the toilet enclosure. Before she retaliated further, the intercom boomed out. "Leave him, we haven't time for this."

"It'll only take me a few seconds."

"Not now. You're injured and thanks to you, he's got a knife as well as that cylinder."

She stood and spat on the floor. "Consider yourself lucky, Ambulance Man."

My heart was thudding as I pushed myself into the corner. I'd worked the blade free from the aluminium tank and was clutching the weapon as if it was my ticket to freedom.

"Why's that, you fucking bitch?"

She dragged a rucksack out from her bunk and threw it over her shoulder before pulling herself up the ladder, her left arm limp against her side. "I never leave loose ends."

"Guess I'm honoured."

"Not for long. You'll be dead soon enough."

The hatch slammed shut, and I heard the spinning sound as the lock sealed me inside.

20

NUTSHELL

Matt reached out a hand to help Tshaarre onto the deck. "Where's the last one?"

She glanced over at the three hooded people sitting in the tinnie. "The paramedic's treating him. He'll have to stay here."

She nodded with her head towards the bridge and the skipper took the hint, motioning her to take the lead. She walked up the stairs cradling her broken arm and once in, he closed the door behind him.

"So what the fuck's going on?"

"Can you get me something to use as a splint?"

"I saw the ambo attack you, but what happened to the other one?"

"He's dead."

"Dead! How?"

"I killed him."

He took the cigar out of his mouth. "What the fuck for?"

"He had inner ear damage that required a hospital."

"So? Still doesn't explain why you fuckin' killed him! You just cost us fuckin' thousands."

"How long do you think it would take them to work out your delivery method when an illegal immigrant turns up in hospital with pressure-related injuries? The paramedic said they're usually caused by diving accidents."

He took a drag from his cigar. "Fuck."

"Yes. Can you get me that splint now?"

He looked about the bridge and grinned, reaching for a thick magazine under the dash. She didn't even flinch as he rolled the publication around her forearm, then used some duct tape to hold it in place.

"There you go, good as new. Thought you'd like Luke's bumper edition Playboy. He won't be needing it and if you get bored, you can look at the pictures."

He laughed and blew smoke in her face. "Now fuck off with the rest of your raghead friends."

His smile dropped as her right elbow jammed into his solar plexus and she launched him back against the wall, pinning him down with her good forearm. Although he could have thrown her aside, the tip of a blade scratching his Adam's apple kept him motionless.

She spoke in a monotone. "You have no idea who you're dealing with."

His larynx bobbed as he swallowed, causing a tiny laceration to weep a tear of blood down his neck. "I was told you were The Travel Agent's bodyguard."

She snorted a laugh. "Tell Fredericks if he thinks I work for The Travel Agent, he's mistaken. The venture capital he received for this little delivery project came with a price. And that price was me."

She pushed herself away from him and, while the skipper rubbed at his neck, she sheathed the knife in a hidden belt around her waist. "Now complete your end of the bargain and get me and my bag out of here."

❋

It was midnight when Bruce returned in the tinnie and Matt was waiting for him on the back deck. "Tell me you've some good news."

"The plane landed on the road, no worries. Got everyone loaded and out within twenty minutes. It all ran like fuckin' clockwork."

"That bitch give you any trouble?"

"No, never said a word. She's fuckin' hot, though. I wouldn't mind bein' balls deep in her."

"Ha. Not a chance, mate. She'd be wearing your balls as earrings before you could crack a fuckin' fat. Now get that tinnie on board while I phone my contact. We've still got some shit to sort out."

Matt climbed up to the bridge and grabbed the sat phone. As he keyed in the number, he glanced at the TV. Three of the images were black, while the last one was a closeup of a jiggling fist, the middle finger raised upright. It disappeared and something squirted on the screen, rendering the fourth square blank.

"Fucking bastard."

A voice came from the phone. "What?"

"Oh… Is the line secure?"

"Wait."

There were a few clicks and buzzes on the line, then Fredericks' spoke. "The scrambler's engaged, go ahead."

"Got some good news and some bad news."

"Good news first."

The skipper relayed the events of the last forty-eight hours, and when he finished, there was silence from the other end.

"You still there?"

"Yes, of course. So, let me see. You not only gave all my

clients the bends, but as a result, one is dead. You've also got your brother's body on your boat and an ambo trapped in the container. An ambo who knows all about our operation. Is that about it in a fucking nutshell?"

Matt's upper lip curled in a snarl. "Yes."

"Well, haven't you created a fucking mess!"

Matt chewed on his cigar while Fredericks contemplated the situation.

After a while, the voice on the line came back. "Fuck it, the risk's too great. Tow the container out deep, then ditch it. We'll use the spare one in Bangkok."

"You sure? I could turn off the pumps and suffocate him."

"And how many tanks of oxygen did you supply him with?"

"There were… Oh, fuck."

"Right. Hit the kill switch and don't fuck up again, otherwise you'll be in the next container that gets dumped."

The connection ended with a click as Matt almost bit through his cigar.

21

PAPILLON

After squirting toothpaste on the cameras, I'd busied myself looking for anything else useful in the bunks. But other than the bottles of protein mix, some tablets and a few phrase books, there was nothing. Sitting on one of the toilets, I tried to think of a way forward, but the hatch only opening from the outside seemed insurmountable. I'd survived the refugees' departure, only to end up trapped like the metal ball inside an aerosol can, and the skipper had his finger on the spray button.

I had one small cylinder of oxygen left, a knife and a few cannulas. Where was MacGyver when I needed him? All the options were with the fucking skipper. He could ditch the container, cut off my air supply, flood the chamber, or bounce dive me a few times so my body fizzed with nitrogen. Any which way I was screwed. The least likely plan would be sending someone in to deal with me, especially as he knew I was armed.

The skipper's voice made me flinch. "Stay away from the

hatch, Ambulance Man. We've got an old friend of yours who'd like to drop in for a chat."

I retreated to the far bunks. Perhaps I was wrong. "Whoever it is, he'd better not enter, if he knows what's good for him."

The skipper laughed. It was a mirthless sound. "Don't worry, he never did know what was good for him."

The hatch dropped open and something large wrapped in plastic was shoved through the hole. About a metre or so was dangling down when the rest fell through and the parcel hit the floor with a thump. A moment later, the hatch slammed shut.

I peered around the corner. Next to Nasim's dead body lay another, wrapped in plastic and duct tape. There was blood and pink goo smeared inside the head end, and as I stretched out the folds to see the face, Luke's sightless eyes stared back at me.

This was not good. There was only one reason for dumping his remains with me: they were using the container as a trash can for all three bodies, mine included. A metal burial chamber that would never be found at the bottom of the Gulf.

As if to confirm my fears, I heard the trawler's engine fire up and the prop start to beat. After a moment there was a jolt as the container's hawsers took the strain and I began being towed out to sea.

I had to think fast.

It wouldn't take them long to get into deep water, but they'd want to make sure they were away from any shipping lanes or fishing spots. What could I do? After the rig released the container, the easiest way to sink it would be to blow the hatch. All that water pouring in would stop me from getting out, but if I waited for it to fill, I could pull myself through the hole.

That said, how fucking deep would I be by then? Could I swim all that way to the surface?

I remembered years ago telling my scuba students how it was possible to swim from depth on one lungful of air, because the gas keeps expanding as you rise. But I'd never used the technique, and the mere notion petrified me.

Then another thought ambushed my mind. What if the hatch didn't blow, and the water seeped in from vents? There'd be no way out. Shit. Think Jono, think!

Panic started to build, and I had to take a moment to calm myself. I sat on the toilet seat again, closed my eyes and focused on the problem at hand, transferring my consciousness to the analytical part of my brain. The anxiety would have to wait.

After a few minutes, my breathing had slowed, and I opened my eyes, looking down at the cylinder by my feet. I could always breathe the oxygen if I was desperate, but that was a recipe for disaster. Unlike being in a chamber, inhaling neat oxygen while diving might cause a seizure, even in shallow waters. At depth, one hundred per cent oxygen would be lethal.

No. That wasn't an option.

I looked at Luke's body and peeled off a length of the duct tape from the plastic and a plan started to form.

The distant pulse of the trawler's prop cutting through the water changed its pitch and almost immediately I felt the pressure building in my head. I grabbed my nose and blew to equalise my ears as we kept descending. Over and over, I had to clear them until the air was thick and condensation dripped from the cold metal walls. They weren't going to make this easy for me.

The intercom crackled into life. "Well, unfortunately for you, we need to be on our way. I've got to get the next fuckin' batch back here in two weeks, so goodbye, Ambulance Man, and thanks for the advice on the bends. I'd like to say it was a pleasure knowing you, but it fuckin' wasn't. Say hi to Luke for me. Tell him his brother still thinks he's a cockhead."

"Fuck you."

"No, Ambulance Man... fuck you."

There was a series of clicks from the walls and the container swayed, as it was released from the rig's stabilisers. Trying to steady myself, I grabbed onto the edge of a bunk as a muted explosion above the hatch caused the cover to burst down, delivering a torrent of seawater. Then something happened that I hadn't anticipated. All the lights went out.

I was plunged into pitch-black darkness as the freezing cold water swirled around my ankles. Light! I needed some light. Without that, how would I find the hatch?

Then I remembered my waterproof pen torch in my top pocket and pulled it out, switching it on before securing the lanyard to my wrist. The beam reflected off the water droplets that were flying in all directions as the sea roared into the room. But the way the container was lurching from side to side was more frightening. It could hit the seabed at any moment and if it rolled over and came to rest on its roof, I was screwed. How could I make sure it went vertical? I could weight one end, but with what?

Surely I wasn't heavy enough... but three of us? I dragged Luke down to the end away from the hatch, bundling him into a lower bunk as best I could. Returning for Nasim, I had to feel around for his body as the water had reached my knees. Once he was installed, I climbed into an upper bunk and waited, flashlight sweeping the room. The level kept rising and just as I thought my idea had failed, the water rushed towards me as the container flipped on its end.

Within an instant, I was underwater and the shock of the cold liquid on my face gripped my chest. I swam upwards through the floating debris and had to kick to stay at the surface. I was above the level of the hatch and could feel the water flowing in, but the rate had slowed, so I took my chance. Holding on to the edge of a bunk, I inhaled several deep breaths before pulling myself along the now horizontal ladder and out through the submerged opening.

The turbulence and speed of the surrounding water told me the container was still descending fast, so I pushed myself away and floated into the black void. Reaching down to my belt, which I'd looped through the handle of the small oxygen cylinder, I cracked open the valve.

Nothing happened.

In a moment's panic, I thought I'd used the punctured tank, and I tried to use the light to see, but the water blurred my vision. Then the plastic bag started to inflate under my arms, and I could feel the water flowing past me as I ascended.

Thud!

An almighty pressure wave hit me that I felt through my body rather than heard. I swung the torch down and could just make out the fuzzy image of the container, standing on its end; sediment billowing out like a rocket about to launch. Fuck! That was close. I may have been able to climb out of the hatch, but there was no way I'd have survived the impact. At least a third of the metal box was crushed and it now resembled a cigarette stubbed into the sand.

I'd made it with seconds to spare, though my trip to the surface was the next huge hurdle. As my balloon inflated I began picking up speed. Despite everything about my being wanting to inhale, the air inside my chest was expanding as the water pressure reduced and so I forced myself to breathe out. From an initial trickle, the escaping air turned into a steady stream as my buoyant ascent quickened. I tipped my head back to ease the flow from my mouth and nose, closing my eyes as the water surged past. Soon I was using all my chest muscles, having to shout to force out the expanding gases. Water buffeted my face and bubbles streamed down my body as I hurtled upwards. By the time I broke the surface, I was screaming like a madman, not just to expel the air, but from the fear of bursting my lungs.

I'd reached such a rate that I shot out of the sea like a submarine missile and was still yelling when I crashed back down. Floundering around, I splashed about, fighting with the huge plastic and duct-taped balloon attached to my belt. It was pinning me down, held beneath the water by the very thing that saved me from the depths. I struggled to release my buckle, fumbling fingers on wet slippery leather, as I felt the edges of my mind clouding from hypoxia. Tendrils of death crept across my consciousness as I willed myself not to suck in any liquid.

Then I was free.

Released.

Sinking.

I kicked hard with a frantic need to return to the living. Seconds later, my face burst from the sea and I took a huge gasping lungful of the beautiful, sweet, cool night air.

I lay on my plastic bag of duct tape and oxygen with my limbs draped over the sides. By some miracle, my makeshift flotation device hadn't ruptured, and it was quite comfortable, lying back soaking wet, staring up at the myriad stars. I felt like Papillon on his raft of coconuts.

Shit, it was good to be alive!

In the first half hour I laughed, shivered, screamed, swore, and wept. In the end, I was just glad not to be on the sea bottom. I thought I'd have at least some barotrauma and kept coughing into my hand, but there were no specks of blood. I must have exhaled long and hard enough to prevent any lung damage. I had a fleeting concern about the bends, but on reflection, my time at depth had been too brief to accumulate nitrogen.

After that, there was a honeymoon period where I revelled in the knowledge I'd survived against the odds. But it wasn't long before reality etched away at my euphoria. I had to face the facts: it was about 2:00 AM; I was lying on a plastic bag that was bound to leak; no one knew where I was; no one was even looking for me; I had nothing to eat or drink; and I was in shark and crocodile-infested waters.

I vowed to myself that if I ever got out of this mess, I'd make that bastard skipper pay. But how? What evidence did I have? It would be my word against his and he was good at covering his tracks. He was off to collect another batch of refugees, and if I blew the whistle, he'd ditch the container. I may have escaped, but I was on my own. It'd be a different story with twenty in that dark, sinking hellhole as it filled with water. Twenty people dead in the blink of an eye. But how could I stop him?

Mind you, whatever I did come up with would mean nothing if I died now. I tried to lift my head to see any land, work out where I was, but I was reluctant to move my position too much. It had taken long enough for me to get on top of the bag.

Eventually I conceded it was too dark, and I was too low in

the water to make anything out. I lay back and stared up at the stars. It was an impressive display. Was it just one day ago when I was looking at them as they took me out to the trawler? Christ, it seemed like a decade had passed. It was a sobering thought that some of those celestial bodies that created those twinkling dots of light billions of kilometres away no longer existed. What was my life in the grand scheme of things when a whole solar system can be snuffed out and few of us even notice?

But how could I waste time on philosophical bullshit? I needed to come up with a plan, devise some solution to my dilemma, quit this quandary. While I thought of what to do, I played with one of my favourite optical illusions, staring at a single bright star. One by one, all the others disappeared, until only the bright star was left. Tiny pinpricks of light, so small the brain dismissed them as background noise when demoted to the peripheral vision.

I woke with an involuntary thrash of my limbs a few hours later, and the movement caused a splash that both confused and frightened me. Recollection flooded into my exhausted mind, and I was both surprised and relieved that I'd managed some sleep. However, I was now cold, aching and felt as if I was wallowing in a paddling pool. Some of the oxygen had leaked from the bag, and my makeshift raft was floating lower in the water.

I lifted my head, and between my feet saw a glimmer of light on the horizon. Off to my right was the low shape of an island, but it was a long distance off. I thought about making a swim for it, but something splashed nearby. There was no way I'd made that noise.

I lay there motionless and waited, straining my ears for the slightest sound. Had it been a wave? I retrieved my pen torch, still on the lanyard around my wrist, and clicked on the button. A beam of light shone out across the water, then retreated into the lens. I guess it wasn't cut out for deep-sea diving after all. But the frustration caused by the loss of my flashlight was nothing compared to the despair spawned by the brief view of my surroundings. Once again, my heart started thudding in my chest. In that moment of illuminated vision, I'd seen at least three fins cutting the surface.

Shit. I willed my body to remain as still as possible and tried to reason with the section of my mind that wanted to scream and thrash about. Look, Jono, you know fish like to hang out under floating objects, right? They're finding a place to chill for the coming day. Fins don't always mean sharks. C'mon, relax, mate. What would swimming do? Just attract the big ones. Hasn't someone shown the splash pattern of a swimmer is the same as an injured fish?

Logic is a wonderful thing, but fear is far more powerful.

I raised myself up as best I could and looked around. Off in the distance, a single white globe swayed above the water. It was an 'at anchor' light. Holy shit, there's a boat over there.

With measured determination, I rolled myself off the plastic, only creating the slightest ripple. I pushed away using a slow breaststroke, keeping my head up and the distant light in front of me. After a few strokes I realised that my work boots were too heavy and would have to go. I retrieved the knife from where I'd wedged it in my shirtsleeve pocket and took a deep breath. Curling up, I reached down and cut both my laces, letting each bulky leather shoe drop into the depths.

When my head bobbed up, the light was gone. I spun around, looking back and forth, then gasped in relief as I spotted it swaying over to my left. Keeping the knife in my hand, I fanned my arms and legs out and continued to perform a slow breaststroke, trying to reduce any turbulence.

Something rough brushed across my bare leg.

Stay calm, Jon! It's just a fish. Only a curious tuna. They hang around floats.

Fuck, their skin's smooth. Sharks have rough skin.

Shit, shit, shit!

I concentrated on keeping my stroke the same rate, not responding, not making a break for it; the last thing I wanted was to look like spooked prey. The light was getting closer and I could see the vague shape of the boat, but it was too far for a dash. Then I realised my nonchalant charade would not deceive a shark. Those pore-like dots all over its nose detected electrical impulses. It sensed heartbeats and mine was pounding.

Thump!

Something hard hit me in the ribs, winding me. This was the first strike, the feint to draw my defence, a test to reveal what risk I posed.

I had to respond.

Had to fight back.

I reached down, blind in the darkness, and felt the dorsal fin. Grabbing the leading edge, I plunged my other hand down, aiming for where the gill slits would be, dragging the knife across the delicate blood-filled structures.

Then I exploded from the water and swam.

Not some tidy, streamlined swimming stroke, but a frenzy of energy powering my body forwards. Gone was the caution. Gone was the pretence. I had injured my attacker, crippling it and creating a decoy, but that blood would attract other sharks in the vicinity. And I couldn't see them coming. No give-away fin steaming my way, no chance to dive to the side at the last second. Just pitch darkness and that goddam swaying light.

The light. It was so near now. I was approaching the back of the boat. So close, but with every pummelling stroke towards safety, I expected to feel the excruciating pain of razor-sharp teeth ripping through my flesh. Five metres. Two. My hands grabbed the duckboard, and I launched myself onto the slatted-wooden platform. Then bang! I was hurled forward and smacked into the transom as something big hit the wood below me. I leapt to my feet and threw my body over the stern, smashing into a wide pole bolted to the deck.

As I lay exhausted on the rough non-slip surface, gasping for breath, I reached out and touched the smooth metal post jammed in my abdomen. My hand contacted the underside of a seat and despite my aches and pains, I laughed. It was a fighting chair, and the only one I knew of in this area was attached to Rob's marlin boat. That current had taken me all the way to Sweers.

One day, when I'm old and grey, I'll sit down and write my memoirs. At that point I might have time to review some of my more pivotal decisions, the ones that had a major impact on my life's direction. The ones that could have gone either way. I'll no doubt spend several paragraphs justifying every one. Why I did this, or why I did that, but the reason for one decision will always stump me. I didn't know at the time and still don't know now why I did what I did after getting on board that marlin boat.

Maybe it was dehydration, maybe it was a desperate attempt to save the next batch of refugees, or maybe it was pure revenge. Whatever it was, in the cold light of day, most would call it insanity.

After banging a few times on the cabin doors, I realised Rob must be staying with the anglers at the resort. Having joined him on a few trips, I knew where he kept his spare key and I made my way around to the bow, reaching under the cradle for the self-inflating life raft. Even in the dark, it didn't take long to find the small waterproof case clipped to the framework.

I climbed up onto the flybridge and started the engine, having to blink as the console of instruments lit up. Once my eyes had adjusted, I checked the fuel tanks were full and weighed anchor, steering the bow north. I knew it was a long shot, but I had to try something. Their trawler would have a top speed of around ten knots, but this baby could manage three times that without breaking a sweat.

I looked at my watch - 5:10 AM. I'd been adrift for less than five hours. At best, they were only fifty nautical miles ahead of me. But Rob's state-of-the-art radar shouldn't have too much trouble picking up a twenty-metre hunk of metal travelling north in open water.

22

MY LITTLE FRIEND

The early morning sunlight streamed into the bridge, as Matt chewed on the stub of his burnt-out cigar and contemplated the radar screen. The blip he noticed earlier had changed direction and was gaining on them. What did it mean?

"You gonna miss 'im?"

"What?"

"Luke. You gonna miss 'im?"

"He was my brother. Of course I'll fuckin' miss 'im. What sorta question's that?"

Bruce shrugged as he sat at the back of the bridge near where Luke's brains had sprayed up the wall. "Just you didn't seem to give a shit when you told me he was dead."

Matt turned to his deckie, who was in his mid-thirties with sandy-coloured sun-bleached hair and a boatie's facial tan, pale patches where his sunnies lived. He was thin, but had a muscular frame. Not from gym workouts, but years of hard labour. He was someone you'd want on your side in a fight.

"There was a lot goin' down that night. I'll deal with it in my own way, in my own time, and not be fuckin' judged by others either way. I've had to watch over Luke since he was born. He was not the easiest kid to like. But he was me brother, and he was family."

Bruce looked down and nodded. "Sorry. I didn't mean to…"

"Look. I know this is not what you signed up for, Bruce, but sometimes shit happens."

He locked eyes with the skipper. "No. You're wrong. I knew exactly what I was gettin' into when I said I'd come aboard. Just didn't think we'd lose one of our own on the first run. I'm not riskin' everythin' for one fuckin' lousy batch of foreigners."

Matt grinned. "Glad to hear it partner, 'cos things might be about to get a bit more serious."

Bruce jumped to his feet. "What d'ya mean?"

Matt pointed at the radar. "Looks like we got ourselves a bogey."

He stared at the display. "You sure?"

"It's travelin' at about thirty knots and coming straight at us. And that's after a course change."

"Boating Patrol?"

"Unlikely from the south and not at that speed. And not a fuckin' chance on a weekend."

His brow wrinkled. "Oz?"

"He would've called me and he doesn't have a boat that travels that fast."

"Who then?"

"Fuck knows, but at that rate, they'll be alongside us in less than twenty minutes."

"So what can we do?"

"Best get ourselves prepared. Y'know that box hidden in the galley I told you and Luke never to touch?"

Bruce gave him a curious look. "Yes."

"It's time to touch it. Go bring it here."

Bruce nodded and loped out of the bridge, sliding down the stairs on the hand rails. He was back a few minutes later with a long wooden box with metal clips securing the top. Matt motioned for him to place it on the map table.

"What's in it?"

"You'll see soon enough."

Matt retrieved a set of keys from his pocket and unlocked the padlock before releasing the catches. He then flipped the lid and cleared away some packing material.

Bruce leaned in. "Wow. What the fuck is that?"

Matt lifted out an olive-green cylinder with white Cyrillic symbols and diagrams on the side. He smiled and said in a bad Cuban accent, "Say hello to my little friend."

The deckie still looked confused. Then Matt flipped up the front sight and extended the barrel, which caused both end caps to open.

"This here's a single-use rocket-propelled grenade. An RPG-22, if you want to be fuckin' precise. They're pretty cheap, if you know where to buy them."

A wide grin broke across Bruce's face. "Fuckin' awesome. It's a bazooka."

23

JUST LET GO

As Sweers disappeared in my wake, I set a course north-east to avoid the rest of the island group and engaged the autopilot. Ducking down to the galley, I raided Rob's well-stocked fridge, guzzling down a couple of litres of water before grabbing some chicken, ham and fruit. Then, after filling a plastic pitcher with juice, I took my bounty back up to the flybridge. The sun was creeping over the horizon as I flew across the waves, and the wind blasting my face helped clear away some of the last remaining cobwebs. Staring at that line in the distance, two simple facts dawned on me: the world's not flat and radars only work by line of sight. I closed my eyes and dropped my head. Shit!

Dredging up a long-forgotten formula from my more active boating days, I launched into some rapid mental arithmetic. Based on my radar's height and that of the trawler, the best range I could hope for was about twelve nautical miles. One look at the chart revealed the distance to the mainland was at least six times that. Finding them would not be easy. Damn! Somehow, I needed to narrow down the search area.

I ripped the flesh off a chicken bone as I mulled over the problem. Their people-smuggling operation must be a day or two behind schedule, and they'd have to make up the time by motoring north. But given their cover as a commercial fishing vessel, I was pretty sure trawlers were tracked, and such a course would look suspicious.

I chewed on the meat and leant back in the flybridge chair, watching the light bleed into the sky, like alkali seeping into a litmus strip. Then it hit me and I threw the bare bone over the side. "Bingo!"

They'll disguise the lack of trawling by heading for a port to off-load their catch. And there's only one north of here: Weipa. I plugged the coordinates into the plotter and set the autopilot for a zigzag pattern to increase the area covered. That done, I turned my attention to the radar screen and waited for the first hit.

It was a long process, but I could discount the initial four pings as they were travelling in the wrong direction, or moving too slow. But the fifth was on the mark. I altered course and began chasing them down.

Until now, my focus had been on the hunt, but if that blip turned out to be them, what the hell was I going to do when I caught up? How could I stop them? Was it possible without endangering myself? Looking at the radar, I had less than twenty minutes to come up with a plan.

The speck on the horizon grew with every second. It was a trawler, but I'd have to do a fly-by to confirm their identity. Keeping at full speed, I hammered past their port side and curved back some distance off their bow, so that my white foaming wake encircled my target. It was them all right.

While still arcing around the vessel, I picked up the radio mic. "Ambulance Man here. Bet you didn't expect to see me again." Without waiting for a reply I called out, "Coast Guard, Coast Guard, Coast Guard, this is..."

But I failed to complete my transmission as I dropped the handset and hurled myself off the flybridge, over the side opposite the trawler.

I'd noticed the skipper appear beside the bridge with a green tube on his shoulder. There was a sudden flame and backblast of smoke, which meant only one thing. I'd underestimated him again.

All I can recall thinking as I plummeted through the air was: where the hell's the water?

Then came the blast.

The missile hit Rob's beautiful watercraft amidships and ripped its way through the gleaming polished hull, dealing a devastating blow, packed with enough power to take down an armoured vehicle. The warhead must have ruptured one of the fuel tanks, as the resulting explosion tore the vessel apart in a huge fireball. As for me, the blast wave picked up my airborne body like a weightless dandelion parachute, throwing me further out to sea.

I tumbled head over heels and bounced twice on the concrete-like water surface before plunging below the waves. My ears were ringing and my lungs burning when I resurfaced, once again gasping for air. I kicked out to tread water and watched aghast as a huge black mushroom cloud rose from the remains of the marlin boat. Due to the speed of the vessel, debris was strewn over a vast area and pieces were splashing down all around me. While I looked on, the smouldering hull keeled over and the sea frothed like a cauldron as it sank from sight.

Through the smoke, off in the distance, I could just make out the stern of the trawler continuing on her way. I hadn't even broken their stride, and now I was truly fucked.

I swam over to a piece of wooden deck that was floating nearby and pulled myself up. My ears were ringing; my head pounding; every bone and muscle in my body was aching, and for some reason my feet felt like they were on fire. Way to go, smart-arse. Another brilliant plan bites the dust.

I lay there for a while, attempting to recover, trying to regain some sort of resolve. But all I could manage was an overwhelming feeling of despair. What was the point? What could I do now? A random wave tipped the deck fragment, and I began to slip back into the water. Perhaps that was the answer.

Just let go.

I'm miles from anywhere, with nothing to drink and no food. No boat. No chance.

Just let go.

Relax, sink down until the air escapes my lungs. Surely drowning was better than the alternatives.

Just let go.

My hands slipped from the decking and I didn't grab out, didn't kick to lift myself back up. I was so tired. It was easier this way. I didn't believe in the afterlife, but if I was wrong, then at least I might meet up with Amber.

Seconds before my head disappeared under the waves, there was a splash and hiss from behind me. In my moribund state, I turned and watched in confused wonder as a bright orange life raft burst from the water and began unfolding in front of me.

24

HELP

"Gonna have to take her higher than usual. See if I can avoid that weather up ahead."

The pilot pointed to some rather ominous looking clouds on the horizon and grinned as he glanced over at his only passenger. "Might make the landing a bit rough, though."

His voice sounded tinny in the bulky headphones Giallo was wearing, and although there was a microphone attached, the detective just nodded.

Somehow he had been convinced to sit in the co-pilot's seat for the eighty-minute charter flight from Mount Isa to Mornington, but he was regretting the decision. The pilot had verbal diarrhoea and had force-fed Giallo his enthusiastic drivel since take-off. Flashing his warrant card had got a discount on the fare, but unfortunately the pilot was into crime novels and had always wanted to be a detective.

Not for the first time, Giallo wondered why people were so discontented with their lot. This one was a pilot for Chrissakes. It would've been far cheaper to sign up to the force. Mind you, a chequered past might have barred his application.

As he prattled on about the plot flaws in his latest read, Giallo appraised him from the corner of his sunnies. He was in his forties, wearing the company-issue white short-sleeved shirt and khaki slacks. His peaked cap and aviator sunglasses covered most of his head, but it was his forearms that intrigued Giallo. Matching intricate tattoos spread from wrist to elbow, depicting extended eagle wings. The fine detail of the shaded blue artwork was impressive, but Giallo couldn't help wonder if their intent was to cover previous prison-made designs.

He sighed and shook his head. Did he always have to think the worst of everyone? As the subject of his deliberations continued to chatter, Giallo felt his way to the end of the headphone cord and pulled the jack out a few millimetres until the audio feed ceased. Silence, apart from the drone from the single prop, but he could cope with that. Now he was at least free to consider the case at hand.

He looked out the side window at the vast expanse of brown parched earth and wondered what chance he had of tracking down his serial killer. Being up here reminded him how big Australia was, let alone the rest of the world. He'd mentioned to Jono that Boardie was like a needle in a haystack. But he was wrong. A sliver of metal in a pile of straw would be far easier to find. And at least the needle wouldn't try to kill him if he got too close.

And what of Jono? Was he dead? Had a croc really dragged him off, or was Boardie to blame? For some reason he couldn't believe the smart-arsed ambo he'd got to know so well had met his end. He guessed that's why he was here with this jailbird pilot.

A blanket of clouds soon blotted out the landscape as they continued to climb to avoid the squall, and a tap on his shoulder interrupted his thoughts. He turned to see the pilot looking at him and shrugged, tapped his headphones and waved his hand.

The pilot reached for the jack and pushed it in. "Huh, your headphone plug came out. I'll have to get that checked. I was asking who's your favourite author?"

"Author? Dunno. I guess whoever writes the ABC news articles."

"C'mon, I mean fiction author. Even a busy detective like you must get time to read a novel or two."

"No. Can't remember the last time I did and if I picked up a novel, it wouldn't be crime fiction."

"Really? Thought you guys would use them for research."

Giallo had to fight the urge not to pull out the headphone cord again. "How long we got left?"

"'Bout twenty. I'll have to start my descent soon. That's when it's likely to get bumpy. So, what d'you need to go to Mornington for? Is it that ambo who's gone missing?"

"Just here for a bit of sightseeing and some fishing."

"Right." He gave Giallo another sideways grin. "Look, no offence detective, but if you ever get offered an undercover assignment you best turn it down."

"Why?"

"Well, if you were here for fishing, you'd have asked me to fly to Birri or Sweers, but you're going to Gununa. And as for sightseeing, let's face it, there's fuck all to see on Mornington."

He laughed, then lapsed into a smug silence, which at least gave Giallo some relief. After a short while, he felt the nose of the plane dip.

"Right, detective, hang onto your lunch. Here goes nothing."

The pilot eased the controls forward, so the plane started a steep descent and swirling layers of water vapour filled their view. The altimeter spun, the fuselage vibrated, and his ears popped. But the windscreen remained white until the clouds gave way to reveal Giallo's first sight of the island. He blinked in disbelief and pushed himself back in his seat. They were coming in at such an angle they appeared to be almost vertical above the runway.

There was a howl from beside him. "Yeeha! Told you it would be hairy."

As they plummeted to earth, Giallo was transfixed by the digits '09' stencilled on the tarmac. Was this it? Was this how his life would end? Staring at the number nine. He let out a small laugh. Wasn't the meaning of life supposed to be forty-two? The pilot pulled back on the steering column and the little Beechcraft Bonanza A36 responded to his commands, flaring into a controlled stall. They alighted on the runway with the lightest touch, then cantered along until their speed reduced to a mere crawl.

With a rev of the engine, he taxied the plane over to the airstrip building and pulled up to a stop. "So, what d'you reckon to that landing, eh?"

"I'll be forwarding you my laundry bill."

The pilot laughed. "They don't call it flying by the seat of your pants for nothing."

Giallo took off the headphones and as he climbed from the plane he called back, "Oh, and for the record, it's Douglas Adams."

"What?"

"My favourite author. Douglas Adams."

As Giallo walked away from the aircraft carrying his duffle bag, a dual-cab ute with police livery pulled up in the carpark beyond the airport apron. A tall Aboriginal man wearing a wide-brimmed Akubra got out and made his way over to meet him.

"G'day, Detective Giallo I presume?"

He held out a leathery hand, and Giallo accepted the welcome. "And you are?"

"Police Liaison Officer Charles Parker, but most people just call me Charlie. I've been assigned as your chaperone while you're on the island, sir. Sorry, I'd have been here earlier, but your plane seemed to drop out of nowhere."

"Tell me about it."

Giallo retrieved a pack of cigarettes from his top pocket and took out a smoke before offering one to his counterpart, who declined. He lit up and enjoyed a deep drag before speaking. "So, Charlie, do I need a chaperone?"

"'Fraid so, sir. You might've been able to pull some strings to get yourself here, but no one's quite sure what you want. You can't be here on official business, otherwise you'd be stayin' at the police station, eh. An' seeing as you cleared your arrival with the Shire Council, they asked me to keep tabs on you." Charlie shrugged. "You're also stayin' at my place, sir."

Giallo finished his cigarette and ground the butt into the dirt. "As I'm here unofficially, you can stop calling me sir. Most people call me Gee."

Charlie grinned. "OK, Gee."

Giallo wiped the sweat from his brow. "Sure hope your place has got aircon, it's fucking hot up here."

Charlie boomed out one of his deep infectious laughs. "Everyone's got aircon up here, my friend. Jump in the cab, it's cool in there, eh. You need to change out of those Brissie clothes. Hope you brought some shorts and thongs."

"Haven't worn shorts since I was in grade ten. Not likely to start now."

He threw his bag in the tray and got in the car, grateful for the kiss of cold air inside the cab.

Charlie reversed the ute out of the parking space. "So, you going to tell me why you're here?"

"If I do, I'll have to shoot you."

Charlie gave a short laugh. "Well, unless you plan on walkin' round town in the swelterin' heat, I'm your wheels. So if you tell me or not, I'll work it out soon enough."

Giallo had to concede he had a point. Whether or not he confided in Charlie was irrelevant, but trusting him now could be beneficial. He'd go with his gut instinct, seeing as this fellow somehow exuded honesty. "OK, I'm concerned about the recent disappearance of your island's ambo, Jonothan Byrne. Something doesn't ring true."

"Glad I'm not the only one who thinks the whole croc story is just that. Y'know, a crock of shit."

Giallo looked at his driver with renewed interest. "So what's your opinion?"

"You first, detective, then I'll tell you what I know. But before that, let's get you installed in my spare room, eh."

They'd pulled up outside Charlie's place, a wooden lowset building raised on posts less than a metre off the ground. It was just along the road from the nursing home and had similar views of the Appel Channel.

Giallo exited the cab and was hit by a wall of heat from the early afternoon sun. "Nice spot. D'you get any cool sea breezes?"

"Usually, but the squall that came through robbed us of 'em. Go take a shower while I crank up the aircon and get a cold drink for ya."

"Sounds good, a beer would go down a treat at the moment."

Charlie laughed. "You want one of them, yous best get

back on that plane. There's no grog on this island. I was offerin' you a soft drink."

"Great. And I guess I have to smoke outside?"

Charlie grinned. "If you don't mind. I'll have you wearin' shorts and down to a pack a day before you know it."

"Ha. Then I will be back in grade ten."

Charlie was sitting at the breakfast table in his kitchen, nursing the remains of a perspiring can of Diet Coke, when Giallo returned from the shower. The detective was wearing an old pair of trainers, narrow-fit blue jeans and a baggy short-sleeved shirt that looked straight from the cheap racks at Big W. His dark black hair was still wet but slicked back, and beads of sweat were already appearing on his skin.

"Feel any better?"

"Marginally. You got that drink?"

"Help yourself, they're in the fridge. There's no full-fat mind, gotta look after me figure, eh."

Giallo picked out an ice-cold can and rolled it on his forehead before sitting down and pulling the stay-tab. He took a few gulps, and the two of them sat in silence.

The detective cracked first. "I guess you're waiting for me to start the ball rolling?"

Charlie grinned. "Us blackfellas know how to wait."

Giallo smiled back and raised his can. "Thanks for the drink. As to why I'm here, I'm sure you know that last year, Mr Byrne exposed a serial killer who'd been operating in Brisbane for some time. The murderer escaped and has so far evaded detection. I'm one of the few still tasked with finding him and when I heard Mr Byrne had disappeared, well, I thought it was worth coming here to check things out."

Charlie grinned. "You're the copper that Jono's been keepin' in touch with, eh. Don't worry, he's told me all about you and the investigation. It's his main topic of conversation. He can be a sad bastard at times, eh."

"Are you deliberately referring to him in the present tense?"

Charlie finished his can. "Well, I don't think he's dead, if that's what you mean. At least, I don't think a croc took him, eh."

"Is that the general opinion here?"

"No. We've got folk out from the Environmental Protection Agency swarmin' over the place, lookin' for Punch."

"Punch?"

"That's what we've dubbed our monster croc. It's a tradition up here to name the big ones. Anyways, most of the locals who can are lookin' as well. Don't get me wrong, there's one out there. I've seen it first hand, but I don't think it took Jono."

"Why?"

He grinned and shrugged. "Look, if you're lyin' drunk on a beach up here, then you're fair game for any croc that finds you, eh. But things don't add up about that night."

"Drunk? I thought you said this was a dry island."

"It is, but there's ways and means." He gave another shrug. "The alcohol laws here are due to this bein' an Aboriginal community, eh. What white folk do on their own is less... scrutinised."

He grinned and fetched more drinks from the fridge, taking a swig before continuing. "We all knew our mate Jono was grievin' and we suspected his drinkin', but he was careful. No one caught him, though no one really tried, eh. It was well known he'd go off on his own with a fold-up table and chair to some remote beach. Next day he'd return lookin' like shit, but as you know, he's got more reason than most to be screwed up."

"So why not that night?"

"Simple. It was a work night, he was on call. Jono never went AWOL when working. He may be a pain in the arse for the ambulance management, but he respects his role and knows the community needs him, eh. In his mind, that fact alone outweighs any personal problems."

"Something could have got the better of him. Maybe a job that day sent him over the edge."

"I've been lookin' into things, eh. That Thursday was pretty cruisy for him; the last call was a false alarm on the headland near Sydney Island. Then nothing until he failed to show on Friday."

"Anyone see him return?"

"No, though both ambulances were in their usual place. Albert lives next to his donga, but he was sick, suffering from a bout of food poisoning, so was dead to the world. And there was a fuss in the hospital 'cos a police dog was recovering in the waiting room."

"A police dog?"

"Long story, but it meant that the duty copper was focusin' more on his mutt that night."

"Still not buying it, but I suspect you've got more."

"One small thing. There's a local lad doin' community service cleanin' the Troopies, y'know the ambulances, eh. Well, he came to me in the arvo to apologise for skipping the inside of one of 'em that morning. He couldn't get in and there was nobody around to give him the keys."

"So?"

"Even though he's had an ambulance stolen, Jono never locks the Troopies. It drives Albert mad, eh."

Giallo shrugged and took a drink from his can. "Keep going."

"Another unusual event that night was the theft of about eight oxygen bottles from the hospital. Might be a coincidence, but it's never happened before and they haven't found the cylinders. The hospital manager's pretty pissed off 'cos they usually just swap the empties for filled ones, eh. Now they're havin' to pay for the missin' hardware."

Giallo tapped his drink can on the table. "I hope you've got more for me to work with than that. You have to admit, it's all a bit thin."

Charlie nodded and scratched his ear. "I know. Nothing but circumstantial shit, eh. I guess if I had something more concrete I'd have presented it to the island police by now. Mind you, there is one thing that has me convinced, eh."

"Go on."

"When I was talkin' to Albert, y'know the Station Officer, he was grumblin' about the drug count being out. The ambos have to record the usage and whereabouts of all the controlled drugs and there's five vials of morphine and five of a sedative called midazolam missing."

Giallo furrowed his brow but said nothing.

"Albert reckons it'll be investigated, but nothing'll happen 'cos the only guy they can ask is dead. They won't want his death linked to lost controlled drugs, eh. Yet here's the thing. He was also goin' on about some other missing drugs, and he showed me Jono's kit. Other than one for sickness, which he uses all the time, there were four different vials gone. Albert couldn't work out why those loops were empty, seeing as Jono hasn't had no jobs that would need 'em since he's been here."

He retrieved a piece of paper from his pocket. "So I got curious and wrote them down." He frowned as he read from the paper. "Serenace, Clexane, Lignocaine, and Phenergan."

Then gave a shrug. "Seeings how I had no idea what they're for, I did a bit of Googling, but nothing made any sense, eh. They're all used for different things. But then I noticed that three of them had two names. It turns out, the ones I copied from the vials were the trade names, y'know, what companies make up to sell 'em. The other name is the actual drug, what Jono's more likely to use. So I noted those down as well, eh. I'd love to say I was smart an' worked it out, but the order I wrote them in was just luck, see."

He handed the crumpled paper to Giallo with the first letters underlined.

Haloperidol.

Enoxaparin.

Lignocaine.

Promethazine.

It took him a second to read the handwriting. Then the detective's eyebrows shot up and his face broke into a smile. "Well, I'll be damned. He made a cry for HELP."

25

LEGEND

Numerous shafts of light spread out from the shimmering disc of gold high above me on the water's surface. They looked like crepuscular rays, the so-called 'fingers of God' created by holes in clouds, diverging outwards like pathways to heaven. It was so peaceful drifting like plankton in the dark blue oceanic water. The sea was cool on my skin and the silence was as comforting as earmuffs on a skiing trip. I was but a speck of dust, suspended like a mote in the beams of light.

Then the need for air forced me to retreat from my sanctuary, return to the surface to refill my lungs. I kicked out and reached up, exhaling as I went, marvelling at the way the light scattered and glistened through the jellyfish-like bubbles rising with me. The sun was almost blinding as my face broke from the water and I took a deep breath. Although the warm air felt good in my chest, I only stayed long enough for a single inhalation before diving back down.

As I swam deeper, I glimpsed a shape moving in the inky darkness of the abyssal depths and stopped my descent. Was it a fish? A shark? A dolphin? It moved with a serpentine grace, keeping itself in the shadows, but circling below me. For a while it stayed too deep to discern any details, but there was nothing threatening in its presence.

Frustrated by my dependence on the air above, I once again had to leave, but was soon back watching the amorphous spectre swirl below me. The shape ventured closer and I could make out the caudal fin of a large fish, but a flowing dark mass hid the head.

Then, with a whip of her tail, she was floating in front of me.

Jet black hair swirled like smoke around her pale white face, and the nipples of her naked breasts stood erect in the cold of the ocean. A smile played across her lips as I tried to scream, thrashing my limbs to escape the inevitable nightmare. Looking up, I saw the distance silhouette of my boat and I kicked hard to reach it, expecting to be pulled down any moment.

But no hands grabbed me and I launched myself onto the transom, wedging my body next to the outboard with my feet dangling in the water. I leant forward, hugging my knees and when I looked up, Amber was watching me, floating nearby.

She smiled. "I thought you wanted to join me, Jon? Weren't you ready to give up and drown yourself, so you could be with me again? Why are you afraid when you're faced with the reality?"

"Reality? This is just another one of my fucked-up nightmares."

"Oh, come on, don't be so hard on yourself. All you need do is swim down to the depths with me. Mind you, you'll have to lose those legs of yours if you want to join me."

She rose up and threw something, which landed with a thud in the outboard's cowling. I looked to see what it was and saw a black throwing knife buried to the hilt in the motor, causing fuel to gush out.

"Ha, missed. You're not as good as Tshaarre."

Lifting a flare gun, she gave me a pitying smile. "Are you sure I missed?"

She pulled the trigger, and the flare ignited the fuel accumulating around my ankles. A sheet of flame engulfed the stern, but I couldn't move, trapped there by my imagination. Scorching agony tore at my feet as I watched my skin blister and burn in the unbearable heat.

Then Amber was beside me in the boat. Her cold wet lips touched my ear and there was a stench of rotting fish as she yelled, "Wake up!"

Consciousness came to me like a rectal exam and an orange world greeted me as my eyes flashed open. I had a moment's panic as I remembered the flames of my dream, but the cold wet sensation against my face and the smell of vinyl brought me back to reality. I was lying on the floor of an inflatable life raft, shaded from the sun by a matching orange canopy.

Moving my head caused the sadist from my hangovers to wield his favourite sledgehammer, pounding my brain into submission. My ears were still ringing from the explosion and I raised my wrist to check the time: 8:30 AM. I'd been out for about forty-five minutes. The slight movement brought on an overwhelming bout of nausea and I pulled myself up on the buoyancy tube to hang out of the entrance.

The fierce pain in my feet was not enough to distract from my vomiting, but as soon as the nausea subsided, I slumped back down and checked them out. Both my soles were red raw with partial-thickness burns peeling away much of the top layer of skin. They'd taken the brunt of the flash from the fireball, and for a second I regretted losing my boots. Then I remembered how close the sharks had been.

I rested my head back on the raft and looked up at the sky. Above me was an immense wall of white water vapour, rolling forward like a cotton wool tsunami. I peered out in both directions and although the huge cylindrical cloud was only a few hundred metres off the water, it extended as far as the eye could see. It was the first time I'd seen the famed 'Morning Glory' roll cloud of the Gulf region, and I wished I could enjoy such a breathtaking spectacle, but the varied pains within my body were too intense. The last thing I remember thinking before I passed out was perhaps the winds that often follow in its wake might blow me closer to land.

Sometimes you have to be careful what you wish for.

I awoke as I was thrown against the opposite wall of the life raft, with the agony in my head and feet causing me to vomit again. I then had to suffer the indignity of rolling about amongst my stomach contents as the plastic floor undulated like a bunch of five-year-olds had been let loose on a bouncy castle. Water came streaming in through the open entrance as another wave hurled me across the raft.

I fixed my arm over one of the grab ropes and zipped down the door, which was thrashing around like a ripped flag in a gale. The brief glimpse I saw of the sky was dark and menacing. No more fluffy white clouds floating on a wash of vivid blue; leaden-grey thunderheads blotted out the sun as they came rolling in.

But that was nothing compared to the sea.

Aggravated by the sudden turbulent storm, fearsome walls of water seemed confused as to which direction to break. Some combined their forces, whereas others crashed in on themselves. White horses leapt in all directions, like in that famous Japanese painting 'The Great Wave' and there I was, helpless as an ice cube in a cocktail shaker.

Although securing the flap had stopped the water flooding in, I was now blind to the next assault, the next spinning swipe, the next yawing blow. All I could do was hold on tight to the rope loops as I was slung around. Without thinking, I used my feet to wedge myself against the side of the inflatable, but the brutal pain firing up my legs put paid to that idea.

As I flopped back and forth, I tried to console myself. Hang on Jono, it won't last long, it's only a squall, ten minutes tops. Then my world turned to shit once again as the raft capsized.

Water flooded into the chamber and I thrashed about to keep my head in the air pocket. When another wave hit, leaving me gasping for air, I realised the raft needed righting. As I kicked to tread water, a long lanyard became wrapped round my legs. Pulling it to free myself, I discovered one end was woven into webbing on the vinyl wall.

A safety line!

I found the free end and fed it through the belt loops of my shorts, tying it off in a bowline.

"Here goes nothing."

I groped my way around the canopy until I felt the door zip and opened it enough so I could slip out. Taking a deep breath, I swam through the hole and into the ocean. It was like diving into a washing machine. The sheer power of the water was astounding, and the first wave whipped me away from the raft. I grabbed hold of the lanyard as it grew taut around my waist and pulled me under.

Working hand over hand, I dragged myself back towards the raft, sucking in a few foam-filled mouthfuls of air on the way. Once at its side, I hooked my arm through a loop and took a breather. Mountains of dark blue water rose all around.

Then a split second later I was skating up a slope and high on a crest, before plummeting back down.

Using the water motion and timing my lunge, I clambered onto the raft's underside and lay there, working out what to do next. Sea spray washed over me and rain stung my face as I looked about. On one edge there was a gas cylinder, which I presumed was used to inflate the craft, and across the middle was a wide strap of webbing material. Not wanting to use my feet, I wedged my knees against the cylinder, raising my body up and pulling on the strap, using my weight to help flip the raft. Try as I may, it wouldn't budge.

"Shit."

I soon realised I would have to stand to get enough leverage, but the mere thought filled me with dread. Then an enormous wave crashed down, almost washing me back into the maelstrom, and the experience fired my animal survival instinct. "C'mon Jono, pain's only your body sayin' you're still alive!"

With that, I leapt up and screamed in both agony and rage. I was like a banshee howling against the wind, pulling with everything I had left. Rain lashed my face as blood pooled at my feet and the strap cut into my hands. One moment I was Ahab fighting the storm, the next I was floundering underwater, submerged in the waves. The cold slapped me from my trance and I kicked out to reach the surface, but just found vinyl. Struggling to hold my breath, I remembered the lanyard and reeled it in, resurfacing by the door of the upright raft.

Coughing and spluttering, I hauled myself aboard and wallowed in the water that had not drained away. Although I was now worse off than when the squall first woke me, it felt so much better and I laughed as the waves sloshed me around the interior. Among the pieces of equipment tied to the inside, I spotted a sea anchor and threw the conical bag out the door, pulling on the line to make sure it deployed. With that simple device set, another capsize was far less likely. Now all I had to do was weather the storm and hope I didn't suffer hypothermia before it passed.

After about half an hour, the buffeting subsided and I could kneel up and use the supplied bailer to scoop out the remaining water. I peered through the opening and saw the sun high in a bright blue sky, the remnants of the storm clouds some distance away. I looked at my watch. It was gone midday. Shit, I must have been out for a good few hours before the squall hit — that'll be the concussion. I sat on the wall of the raft, hanging onto the canopy, and searched the horizon.

Nothing. Other than sea and sky.

"Guess there's no point callin' for an ambulance."

I laughed, but soon realised I was trying to stop myself from crying. Once again, I had to face the facts. I was on a tiny orange dot in the middle of nowhere, with no water or food. And the capsize had tainted any rain that had collected in the canopy. But hey, I could look on the bright side. At least there wasn't a Bengal tiger with me; I reckon its claws would have made short work of the vinyl raft.

With no land in sight, I thought I'd better take stock of what I had. I slipped back onto the wet floor, being careful not to catch my feet, and pulled out the tied-down watertight equipment bag. One of the first things I spotted was a three litre sealed bottle of drinking water. Now there was a start. But as I rummaged through the usual items, like flares, a paddle, a flashlight and puncture repair kit, a small black pelican case grabbed my attention. I dried my hands as best I could and flipped open the catches.

Inside, nestled within matching foam cutouts, was a satellite phone, spare batteries and a dedicated solar charger.

I closed my eyes and thanked the raft's owner. "Rob. You're a fuckin' legend."

With reverent care, I lifted out the phone and pressed the red 'on' dial. Nothing. I held down the button. Nothing. I flipped over the satphone and pushed off the battery cover, slotting in a spare. Still nothing.

All the batteries appeared dead. "C'mon Jono. Don't be a cockhead, read the manual."

I did, and it confirmed they were dead. "Shit."

Step by step, I followed the instructions to charge the batteries, opening the raft's door and positioning the two clamshell-like panels on top of the dry case to pick up the most light. After that, I was dismayed to see the small print: Please note, it may take two or three charging cycles to charge a flat battery.

"Great. How long's a fucking charging cycle?"

Presuming I was in for a few hours wait at the very least, I made myself as comfortable as possible and read the satphone manual from cover to cover. Other than being able to call anyone's phone number, it could also send texts and transmit your GPS coordinates. Cool.

Although my feet were still hurting, there was nothing in the small first aid kit to treat them, so I gave up on that idea. The pain had eased a lot, anyway. Instead, I sat and watched the blue light on the charger blink and thought about who I would phone first.

But my dilemma had not changed. If I called in the authorities, twenty refugees would likely perish. And what actual evidence did I have regarding their operation? How could I prove any of my claims? Without hard facts, Oz and the trawler men would go free. They had more on me for stealing

Rob's marlin boat than I had on them for people smuggling. After all, I'd disappeared from work and now I was sitting in his life raft.

To ensure a conviction, the bastards would have to be caught in the act and the police or immigration officials would take a lot of convincing to allow a risky venture like that. All on the say-so of a burnt-out ambo.

The heat and humidity built inside the canopy as the sun's rays evaporated the water. In response, I fashioned a clothes line from the safety lanyard and stripped naked, hanging out my things to give them and myself a chance to dry.

After a while, a second charger light began flashing, and I took a swig from the water bottle to celebrate. Then another thought struck me. Even if I could convince the authorities to launch a sting operation, how would I hide my own rescue? If the coastguard picked me up, the event would be plastered all over the news. Missing ambo found adrift. Especially if they dredged up my serial-killer connection. There'd be no point in waiting for the skipper to smuggle in his next batch of paying customers. He and Oz would be off like a bucket of prawns in the sun.

No. I needed someone to come and pick me up on the down low and help me catch all the bastards red-handed. There I was, feet burnt to a cinder, lying stark naked in a life raft, lost somewhere in the vast expanse of the Gulf, and a smug smile crept across my face. I knew just the man for the job and what's more, I knew his phone number.

26

SEASICK

"Christ. Are all the roads like this?"

Giallo had been hanging onto the passenger grab handle ever since they left the sealed streets of Gununa. After some discussion, the two of them had decided to check out the location of Jono's last call. It seemed as good a place to start as any.

Charlie let the back end of his dual cab slide a little as he guided the vehicle round the next bend. Grinning, he turned to Giallo. "You should see 'em in a month or so's time, eh. Can't use 'em at all when the wet season sets in proper."

The rain from the brief storm that lashed the island prior to the detective's arrival had mixed with the loose dirt on the road's surface, converting it to a layer of mud. But at least the water hadn't penetrated too deep, and the tracks were still passable.

Giallo scanned the terrain. A flat landscape littered with short scrubby bushes stretched out in every direction. The uniformity was punctuated by the odd tree that stood proud from its diminutive cousins, like a weed on a manicured lawn.

"Does anyone live away from the town?"

"Some folk have houses near the sea."

"So how'd they get about the island in the wet season?"

"They don't. Most return to Gununa. The only way of getting supplies is by your own boat, unless you stock up for several months. And livin' off tinned food ain't my idea of fun."

Giallo gave him a sly look. "Can't you live off the land any more?"

Charlie laughed as he swerved to miss an exposed rock. "Bush tucker's fine for survivin', but I prefer livin', eh."

They bounced and slid the rest of the way with minimal conversation until they pulled up at the beach where the road petered out. Charlie stepped on the brakes and they came to a crunching halt.

"Well, that was a roller-coaster ride. I didn't realise we were in such a rush."

"Bit rough for a city slicker, eh? Seriously, if you go too slow on these roads you'll end up getting bogged."

Giallo peeled his aching body from the passenger seat and jumped from the cab, instantly regretting leaving the aircon so soon. Then again, he needed a smoke. He lit up and stepped onto the sand, despising the humidity, but enjoying the nicotine hit.

Waves, dirty with churned-up sediment, crashed against the shore as the energy from the distant storm still exerted its influence on the water mass. A low island lay about two kilometres off to their left, but other than that there was little to report. Charlie came out to join him and squatted down on his haunches near the strandline, looking up and down the beach.

"Not much here, eh."

"What's that island?"

"We call it Langunganji, but you guys named it Sydney Island."

"Bit easier to say."

"Maybe for you."

"So what the hell was Jono doing here?"

"A report from a boat reckoned they could see a ute rolled over on the land."

"Does he usually get sent out to stuff like that?"

"Depends. Sometimes. Plus Miles, the island's copper, was busy looking after his dog."

"Right."

Giallo took another drag from his cigarette. "So, read out that transcript again."

Charlie had written down the recording of Jono's last conversation. He pulled out a notepad and flipped through the pages. "Here it is: Hi, I'm out at the location you gave and there's nothing in this. I've searched the beach all along the headland. The only thing I found was some bleached driftwood and a couple of washed-up old tyres. I guess that's what they saw. If it's OK with you, I'll start the long return back to station."

He put the notepad away and looked up at Giallo.

"Did he sound his normal self?"

Charlie paused for a moment. "No. Not his usual cocky self."

Giallo frowned as he took another drag on his cigarette. "How far does he cover?"

"Jono? Well, for most of the time there's only one ambo for the whole of the Wellesleys, but nearly everyone lives in Gununa. Why?"

"How big's the island?"

"Oh, 'bout seventy Ks."

"Why would he say 'long return back to station'?"

Charlie shrugged his shoulders. "Dunno."

Giallo slapped his forehead. "Oh shit."

"What?"

"It's another one of his fucking alphabet clues. Long Return. LR. It means Law Required. Yet another fucking cryptic cry for help."

"Shit. He was hopeful, eh."

"What d'you mean?"

"Well, that his Comms would work that out. He must have been clutchin' at straws. He says they couldn't work out a turd from their own arse."

Charlie's ringtone playing from his pocket interrupted their laughter. He retrieved his mobile and took the call. "Miles, what's up?"

Charlie stood and paced a few strides as he listened to the caller. "Really, what, Doc Marsh? Y'mean that big expensive thing? Shit. No. Haven't heard anythin'. I'll put m' feelers out. See what I can find for you, eh. No worries, mate. I'll be in touch."

He put his phone away and shook his head.

"Another weird thing happen?"

"No, well, maybe. Someone stole a boat, eh."

"Not that unusual, then?"

"It is for around here. The boat's worth a fortune, and we all know it belongs to one of our doctors. None of the locals would screw with it."

"When did it go missing?"

"This mornin'. It was moored over at Sweers Island. That's about fifty Ks that way." He pointed to the south-east. "Problem is, the Doc can't get back. He's stuck over at the fishing resort until he can arrange a charter flight."

"You've got a resort up here?"

"Yep. It's Disneyland for fishermen. I could think of worse

places to be stranded. It's got the only bar between here and Burketown."

Giallo stared in the direction Charlie had pointed. "Fifty kilometres you say."

"You'll never make it. Sharks'll have you if the crocs don't."

He shrugged. "Well, let's get back to business. Can't see any washed-up tyres on the beach and if he was trying to call LR, that means the rest of the message..."

A chime from Charlie's phone interrupted him, and Giallo frowned.

"Sorry, I'll switch it off."

"Anyway, I'm guessing what he said was made under duress. But why here and what for?"

Charlie was staring at his phone screen. "What the fuck..."

"Bad news?"

He held up his hand. "Hold on, I just got a text... Is it some sorta hoax? I've got to take the next call."

Giallo flicked his spent butt and lit up another as he walked out onto the beach, pondering his own questions. Then he heard Charlie's phone start ringing.

"Oh my God, it is you! Hey, hey, it's so good to hear your voice mate, where are you?"

The detective blew smoke in the air. "Are you always this popular?"

He turned to see Charlie's face beaming with a wide smile. "Actually, Gee, you need to take this, otherwise you won't believe me."

I managed to charge another satphone battery before the light faded. I'd arranged with Charlie to transmit my location every thirty minutes, so the last thing I wanted was to run out of power. He'd called at about 5:00 PM to say they were on their way and their satnav reckoned it would take about five hours, if they could maintain twenty knots. At the time, I'd looked out at sea and was amazed how fickle the Gulf could be. One minute I was hanging on for dear life amid a squall and the next it was gradual undulations, a wave pattern you'd be hard-pressed to see on an oscilloscope. Now back in my almost-dry clothes, I was being treated to a glorious sunset. A smouldering, fiery globe dissolved into the calm horizon like an inverse vitamin tablet, colouring the air orange instead of the water.

As the dark closed in, I noticed a few fins cutting the surface nearby, but this time they were only tuna finding a place to spend the night. I did consider whiling away the hours with some fishing using the supplied hook and line, but the risk wasn't worth it. Combining hooks, a pissed-off fish, and an inflatable was asking for trouble. A day without food was better than losing the raft.

So I just lay there, trying to get comfortable. My feet were still hurting, but the pain had reduced to a dull ache, so long as I didn't move them. Earlier, I'd made the mistake of flexing my big toe and the taut burnt skin beneath split and began bleeding. I guess my ballet career was over.

Soon it was pitch dark, apart from the intermittent bursts of light coming from the automatic strobe fitted to the raft. The only noise was the lapping of the water against the side. I was exhausted, but I had to stay awake to send my location. Plus, sleeping held the threat of another Amber visit, so I spent the time thinking of how I could trap the people smugglers.

The plane's arrival was their obvious weak point, but if I'd identified that, then I could assume they'd have countermeasures in place to protect the vulnerable part of their operation. I thought for a while about what they might do to mitigate the risk, then it dawned on me. The plane itself. It arrives at night, so they could have an infrared thermal camera to assist with landing. Technology like that would show up any heat signatures nearby, such as authorities lying in wait. One sortie would reveal any boats, vehicles, or people hiding in the vicinity. If anything seemed suspicious, they could simply fly off and the trawler would leave and dump the cargo. No evidence. A clean getaway.

The more I considered the possibility, the more convinced I became that a thermal imager was their solution. Either way, any plan to catch them would have to take that into account. I looked at my watch and the fluorescent dial glowed at me in the staccato darkness. Shit, it was still only 8:23 PM.

After seven minutes, I sent another text with my GPS location, then relaxed against the inflatable wall to mull over my situation. A moment later, my thoughts were interrupted by a slight noise coming from the other side of the raft. I reached for the flashlight I'd secured to my wrist and flipped it on to see Amber staring back at me.

She held her hand in front of her eyes. "Ooh Jon, that's bright, switch it off, would you?"

Her long, dark hair was soaking wet and hung close to her pale skin. I was not game to discover if she was still sporting a tail, so did as she asked and switched off the light. "Shit, I've fallen asleep again."

"What, you're not glad to see me any more?"

"Just fearful of the next thing my fucked-up subconscious has in store."

She dropped her mouth open, mocking me. "That's no way to speak to a lady."

"You ain't been acting like a lady, Amber."

With every pulse of the strobe, I could make out the shape of her body, projected as a silhouette on the orange backdrop.

"Look, Jon, I've got to attract your attention somehow. Get my message across. Like now. Why do you need to catch these guys? Can't you just let the authorities know what they're up to? Leave the police to deal with it. Do you always have to play the hero?"

I sighed. "It's not about being a hero. If I blow the whistle, then twenty refugees will die. You of all people should understand. The last time I blew the whistle I lost you. I don't want any more lives on my conscience."

"But these guys have tried to kill you twice already. Three times if you count that green-eyed woman. Your luck's going to run out sometime."

"My luck ran out when that knife entered your chest. Yours wasn't the only heart that was ripped open that day."

"Oh come on. Don't get so melodramatic with me. We were managing a rational discussion. You don't want me to do something weird to frighten you again, do you? Shock you back to the world of the living?"

I let out another sigh. "Sometimes I think the world of the living is over-rated. But no, Amber. I never want to fear you, and I will move on. You'll always be with me, in my memories, and it was a privilege to have known you. You're right. I've been moping around up here, and I've decided to go back to Brisbane, restart my life. But I have to sort this mess out first."

The raft wobbled with her shifting weight, and I felt the warmth of her body next to mine. I flinched despite myself, expecting some abomination to befall me from another horrific hallucination, but she rested her head on my chest. I could smell the sweet, familiar scent of her hair and draped my arm around her shoulders.

She shrugged. "OK. Catch your bad guys, but promise me you'll be careful."

As I hugged her, I felt a salty tear trace a path down my face.

"Of course I will."

"Well, I guess you'll be needing this then."

She placed something in my hand and in the dim rhythmic light I could see it was the satphone. As soon as I focused on it, the device rang.

I opened my eyes and looked around. The shrill tone of an incoming call was deafening in the confines of the raft. Shaking my head, I grabbed the phone and pressed the green pickup button.

"Uh-huh?

"Hey Jono, you fall asleep?"

I glanced at my watch, 10:19 PM. "Maybe, what's up Charlie?"

"Well, we're near the GPS fix of the last coordinates you sent, but we can't see you. Any chance of sending up a flare, eh?"

"I'd rather not fire one into the sky for all to see, but give me a second and I'll light a handheld for you. Plus I'm sending my current location now. See ya soon."

"Lookin' forward to it, mate."

I cut the call and transmitted the data before flipping on the flashlight and grabbing a flare. Ducking through the door, I knelt on the inflatable's wall and ignited the device, holding it as high as I could. From the moonless dark, an intense light burst from the stick, surrounding the raft in a dome of illumination that caused me to squint.

The blaze lasted for thirty seconds, before fizzing and spluttering to a stop, so I slipped back inside and called Charlie's number.

"D'you see that?"

"Yep. You're still some distance off, but we can now see your strobe. We'll be with you in five."

"Cheers."

No longer worried about conserving the batteries, I hung the flashlight from the loop inside the canopy and it swayed in the gentle swell as I lay there with a smile on my face. Rescued within fifteen hours. The land of the living never looked so good. I'll have to thank Rob for his foresight, that's presuming he'll ever forgive me for losing his boat. The night was so quiet and I strained my ears for the sound of the approaching engine, but nothing.

Just as I had my doubts, I picked up the distant whine of their outboard. I switched off the phone and returned it to its waterproof case. It was a handy device to keep with me, but the raft would have to go. There could be no evidence I survived the boat's sinking.

The noise was getting louder, and I looked out the door to see a cone of light coming my way. I gave them a wave and lifted myself up onto the inflatable's wall. The boat pulled alongside, with Charlie's white teeth gleaming in the torch beam.

"Hey, Jono. You lookin' for a lift?"

I grinned at him. "'Bout bloody time you showed up, I was just thinking about swimming back. Hey, you OK, Gee?"

The detective was wearing a very serious expression and appeared pale in the artificial light. He held up one hand with the palm out, while the other gripped the edge of the boat. Then he leaned over the side and vomited.

Charlie rolled his eyes. "He started that when we were still at the jetty. He's not so bad when we're motoring, but as soon as we slow down he chucks. I'm amazed he's got anythin' left to spew, eh."

Giallo wiped his face with his hand. "Can you just get in the fucking boat so we can return to land?"

"Anything you say Gee. You have no idea how good it is to see you guys."

Charlie reached over and pulled the raft in close. "There's a blanket, water, and some food in the dry bag there."

"You're a lifesaver, literally."

As I swung myself into the boat, taking care of my feet, Giallo sat back on a bench and lit a cigarette.

Charlie frowned. "Probably not a good idea, Gee, you bein' near the fuel tank 'n'all, eh."

Giallo gave Charlie a glare and took a deep drag, holding onto the smoke better than his stomach contents. As he exhaled, he looked my way. "What happened to your feet?"

I sat on the seat next to him and opened a bottle of water, guzzling some down before answering. "It's a long story. I'll fill you in on all the details when we get back, but I'm sure you don't want to bob around here while I ramble on."

"I guess I can wait."

Charlie looked at us. "What 'bout the raft. Leave it, bring it, or sink it?"

"Sink it. Don't want any chance of it being found. They think I'm dead and we need to keep it that way."

"They?"

"Part of that long story."

He nodded and unclipped a utility knife from his belt, spinning the raft around and ripping a large hole in each of the flotation chambers. I looked on with mixed feelings as I watched the vessel that had saved me from a watery grave sink below the waves, the flashlight and the strobe illuminating its decent into the depths. I pulled the blanket over my shoulders, more for comfort than warmth, and chomped a grateful bite out of a hunk of chicken. It was from the Gununa convenience store, but it tasted as if it was from the Savoy.

Giallo took one look at me and spun round, retching over the side.

In between mouthfuls, I apologised. “Sorry, Gee.”

Charlie and I shared a grin as he put the engine in gear.

“Whose is the boat, Charlie?”

“Me uncle’s. I told him I was going to search for the croc that’s supposed to have taken you.”

“So that was their cover story.”

“Cover story or not, there’re loads of people searching for you and he was more than willing to help, but I got to return it tonight, eh. He needs to check his crab pots in the mornin’. Pull your head in Gee-man, we’re about to speed up. The journey back won’t be as far. I’m gonna drop you guys off at a place I know on the north end of the island.”

He pushed the throttle forward and the twin outboards behind me responded with a low grumbling roar, lifting the boat onto the plane. The only light was from the satnav, which painted Charlie’s face in a dim glow. He had dropped everything to come to my rescue, with little to explain how and why I was floating on a raft in the middle of nowhere. And as for Giallo, I could just make out his shape, leaning back on the bench next to me. Even his outline appeared to be suffering. He must have known he’d get seasick before he left to look for me.

The wind whipped across my face, and I smiled as I looked up at the twinkling stars. At that moment I realised I was in the company of two men I could honestly describe as true friends.

It was gone 1:00 AM when Charlie eased off the revs and the boat came down off the water's surface. Despite the blasting wind and buffeting motion of the waves, I'd spent most of the journey huddled on the bench seat, asleep. When I awoke, my night vision picked up two silhouettes talking at the helm.

"I'll drive us straight up the beach, so you can jump out onto the sand. Wouldn't want you to get your trainers wet, eh."

Giallo stood up. "Wet or dry, I'll just be glad to be back on land."

"Once there, if you steady the boat by holding the anchor line, I'll join you and help haul it up, eh."

Charlie turned towards me. "Oh hey, look. Sleepin' beauty's awake. We're here, Jono. You able to give us a hand?"

"Hand yes, feet no. I can crawl, but I can't walk, especially on sand. My feet are going to need some work."

"Shit. Right. Any ideas how we're going to get you to the house, eh?"

I shrugged. "Piggyback?"

Charlie looked at Giallo, who returned the stare for a few moments, then twisted around and vomited into the water.

"Guess that'll be down to me, eh."

He shook his head and drove towards the beach, raising the outboards at the last minute and coasting in on a wave. There was a shushing noise as the keel cut into the sand and we came to a gradual rest. Then he stepped up over the bow and jumped down.

"C'mon Gee-man. Stop your spewing, there's land over here."

Giallo made another attempt to stand, but a wave bumped the boat, and the uneven weight caused the vessel to lurch over. Giallo went head over heels overboard in a neat somersault, landing on his backside with an enormous splash.

Charlie's laugh boomed out across the deserted beach and I called out between my own laughter. "You said wet or dry, mate. Didn't think you were that keen to get on land."

Giallo stood up in knee-deep water and used a hand to comb his hair while blowing a drip off his nose. "Well, that was fucking refreshing."

Then he made a desperate grab for his top pocket. "Hey, look at that. Neither my phone nor my smokes got wet."

He waved the pack at us to prove his point and lit up a cigarette as he waded out of the water. "Right. So where's this house? I could do with a bit of shut-eye, once I've dried off."

"Well, stop clowning around and help me make the boat safe, then we'll go find it."

They pulled the vessel a few metres up the beach, and Charlie threw out the anchor before grabbing two flashlights. "Right, Jono. You sit tight, we'll be back soon. I'm not carrying you any further than I have to."

"No worries."

I watched as their light beams wandered up the shore and into the undergrowth past the strandline. Then I was once again on my own, but this time without the fear. I relaxed and watched the stars, wondering if any solar systems had been snuffed out since this whole shit fight began.

I woke to the sound of their approaching voices and looked up to see the flashlights waggling along the beach like a pair of demented fireflies in a grey-shaded landscape.

"Find it?"

"Yep. It's about four hundred metres that way. It'll be a hike with your lard-arse on me back, but not impossible."

"Just be glad I ain't your mother."

Charlie laughed. "You ain't met me mother. She's half your size and would beat the crap out of you for just suggestin' she's fat. You're a brave man, Jono, for bringin' her into it."

"Mmm... Brave. Don't think that's the word I'd use. Anyway, let's get out of here."

I swung my legs over the side and Charlie knelt down so I could climb onto his back. He then stood and adjusted my position.

"Shit Jono, you weigh a tonne, eh."

"Bout eighty kilos, but it's all lean muscle."

Giallo was now holding the dry bag and both flashlights. "Bet fifty kilos of that's in his head."

"Don't make me laugh, I might drop 'im, eh."

We were all still laughing as we started up the beach, with Giallo's shoes squelching every step.

As we left the sand, I looked around. "Where the fuck are we, Charlie?"

"This headland's known as Nyuldora. We're on the north-east side of the island. 'Bout as far away from anyone as possible, eh."

He stopped to take a rest. "The White Cliffs are about two Ks that way."

He nodded his head to indicate the direction and carried on walking. After a while, I snorted out a laugh.

"What's up?"

"Guess you've now got proof that white fellas ride your arse."

"You keep makin' me laugh and your lily-white arse will be crawling to the house."

Giallo joined in. "Just a warning, Jono. The term 'house' is a little misleading. Shack would be more accurate."

"Anything's better than that raft."

"True. Anything's better than any fucking boat if you ask me."

"I'm amazed at how much spew you chucked, eh. I'm surprised you weren't throwin' up y'own shit."

"Tasted like I was."

The banter died down until Giallo spoke. "Talking of that raft, you able to tell us what the hell's going on, now I can hear myself think?"

My mind still felt groggy, almost punch-drunk. "When we get inside. Suffice it to say, you can't trust anyone at the moment."

"Why not, eh, Jono?"

"Let's get inside first."

We carried on trudging through the undergrowth in silence until the flashlight illuminated a lowset brick building that looked like it hadn't fared too well during the last cyclone. Or perhaps a few before that. I could see a large crack spreading across one wall, a window was broken, and the nearby vegetation appeared to be trying to reclaim the land. But although the roof seemed tattered, it was intact and for me, it held the promise of a dry bed.

"Get the door, would you Gee."

Charlie lumbered inside, bouncing me off the walls as we walked down a corridor and into a bedroom. I rolled off his back and flopped onto a small single bed. A cloud of disturbed dust sparkled in the torch beam, and there was a strong musty smell. But it was dry. And it was soft. And my life was no longer in immediate danger. Exhaustion enveloped me as if I was sinking into quicksand and I only just registered a voice asking a question before I descended into a blissful, dreamless sleep.

Charlie and Giallo looked at each other. "Guess we'll have to wait 'til he wakes to know what the fuck's goin' on, eh."

27

OZ

I woke to the smell of cigarette smoke accompanied by a throbbing headache. Attempting to open one eye caused more pain, so I opted to listen for a few moments, see if I could get my bearings by sound alone. The sea nearby was rolling to the shore, but closer was a creak of wood and the slight wheeze of air flowing through nasal passages. The mustiness of the mattress brought my recollection flooding back, and I stretched my body, feeling for the aches that I knew would come.

"'Bout time you woke up. Not much to do here except smoke and sweat."

I rolled over and propped myself up on my elbows. There was a ray of light emanating from a closed pair of faded curtains, which dissected the room like a shaft of gold slashing the darkness. The creaking noise came from a dark form in the room's corner. I could just make out the shape of a man rocking back on a chair. The tip of his cigarette flared as he inhaled a breath.

"How long you been there, Gee?"

"Few hours. It's the coolest part of the house, which ain't saying much."

"What time is it?"

"About midday. You've been sleeping like a baby. Didn't have the heart to wake you, but I do have a few burning questions I need answering."

"Don't suppose there's any coffee?"

"Just a tick. I'll call room service and get you a full English brought up."

He took another drag on his cigarette. "No, the best I can offer is a bottle of water and a few Oreos, though they're a bit stale. I'm hoping Charlie'll bring some more supplies."

I blinked a few times and yawned, looking around. "Where is he?"

"He had to return the boat. He'll have needed a few hours' kip before braving the drive out here. We'll be lucky if he turns up before nightfall. Plenty of time for you to tell me what the hell's going on."

"Got that water?"

"Catch."

A plastic bottle came flying out of the gloom, and I caught it just before it hit my face. "Thanks, I think."

"C'mon. Enlighten me. Are we dealing with Boardie?"

"Ha! If only." I cracked the lid and took a mouthful. "One serial killer would be easy to deal with compared to these bastards."

I reached up and opened the curtain so I could see the detective, then dragged my body up the bed to lean on the wall. The bright sunlight hurt my eyes, but I needed to watch his reaction when I told him the story. I then embarked on a blow-by-blow account of all that had happened since saving the police dog's life. At the end, Giallo was silent.

"Any more water?"

"There's plenty in the tap, but Charlie warned me not to drink it, unless I wanted my arse to spew like me on a boat."

"That paints a vivid picture." I rubbed my forehead, wishing the headache would ease. "So what d'you reckon to my story?"

"Sounds like you were lucky to escape with only your feet being barbecued. Why can't we just call in customs or the navy?"

"We could, but the smugglers would dump the container. Apart from the loss of life, it'd be difficult to prove they were towing it, even if they were able to retrieve the bodies. And that could take weeks."

"They can do undercover stings, you know. Some of us cops are quite good at that sort of stuff."

"Yes, but on an island like this? Everyone knows everything that goes on here. How d'you propose they get a team anywhere near here without Oz catching wind of it? And that's presuming he's the only one involved. Their setup must be worth a fortune. How'd we know no one else's being paid to look the other way, or worse still, supply information?"

Giallo remained silent as he lit up another smoke.

"I presume Oz already knows there's a detective over here. Even the chance that he does means we'll have to come up with a cover story for you."

Giallo leant forward so the chair landed on all four legs and then combed a hand through his hair. "Well, if he thinks I'm here to investigate your disappearance and wants to get rid of me, what he needs to do is simple."

"Which is?"

He blew out a cloud of smoke and shrugged. "Make a big show of finding the croc that ate you."

❧

It was midday when Charlie drove his dual cab into the Gununa fuel station and pulled up at the bowser. He'd raided his place for supplies and called in to the grocery store for fresh food, which he packed in the esky now strapped in the ute's tray. His last stop was to fill a jerrycan for the generator, plus he had to refill and return the ones used on his uncle's boat.

He was still pouring petrol into a large red marine tank when a ute stopped at the other bowser. There was a loud creak from the door as Oz climbed out. He tapped the peak of his hat before unscrewing his own fuel cap.

"Charlie."

"Oz."

The fisherman's face wrinkled in a scowl as he looked at the container Charlie was filling. "What you doin' in a boat, Charlie? Thought you stuck to the jetty for your fishin'."

"Ah, borrowed me uncle's boat, eh. Wanted to do my bit for Jono, y'know, see if I could find Punch. If he's the one that took him."

Oz slotted the nozzle into his ute and started pumping fuel. "Any luck?"

"Drove all the way round the island with a flashlight. Only found little-uns, but. Nothin' that could drag a fully grown man down a beach. I think this whole serial-killer croc sounds like bullshit, eh."

"Bullshit? That ambo's nothin' but crocodile shit by now. Sorry, Charlie... no offence. Know he was a mate of yours 'n'all. But he ain't been seen for three days. What else coulda happened?"

Charlie shrugged. "Guess I just don't wanna believe it."

"Yer, fuck of a way to go."

He loaded the tanks into the ute while Oz hooked up the hose he'd been using and they both walked towards the shop. "Heard you're babysittin' a cop from the big smoke."

Charlie smiled and gave another shrug, but said nothing.

"Oh, I get it. Official police business." He pushed open the door and a metallic buzzer went off as they entered the aircon. There was no one behind the counter, so they stood and waited.

"Your city cop here looking for the croc as well?"

Charlie turned to Oz. "You seem to be askin' a lot of questions today, eh."

"Need to keep tabs on my competition. That croc's worth a shitload to me. I've already got the EPA officials breathin' down me neck. Anyway, didn't mean anything by it. You go have a good campin' trip, mate."

Charlie grinned, realising Oz had checked out his ute. "Perhaps you should be the detective, Oz." He then leant towards him, lowering his voice. "Between you and me, that cop wouldn't make the water police. Spewed all night. We now gotta search from the land. If you ask me, he ain't got much clue about crocs."

Oz frowned. "So why the interest?"

Charlie shrugged. "He was a friend of Jono's."

A rotund man came in from a side door, wiping his hands. "Charlie. Oz. Sorry to keep yous waitin', just in the dunnie. It's typical, sit here for hours, but soon's I leave to take a leak, two o' yous show up. So, who's first?"

Oz stepped back and waved a hand. "After you, Charlie."

Charlie paid with cash and said his farewells, but as he walked from the shop, he overheard the attendant. "That'll be five twenty, Oz. Jeez, last of the big spenders, today, eh."

Sweat trickled down my neck and bathed my forehead. The heat was becoming oppressive, but moving elsewhere in the house would be difficult, and Giallo had said this was the coolest room. I looked up and spotted an archaic rusty split system above my head.

"I presume the aircon isn't working."

"No, it works fine, we're just out of electricity. We need to get some fuel for the genny, which is another thing that Charlie's bringing."

He moved his weight on the chair. "A change of clothes would be nice. My jeans are as stiff as a board after that dip last night."

"Don't have to tell me. There's so much salt in my shirt and shorts I reckon they could stand up on their own."

I wiped the sweat out of my eyes and considered drinking the dodgy tap water. "So… Now you know this whole mess is nothing to do with Boardie, are you going to hang around and help catch the bad guys?"

Giallo didn't respond while he savoured his last cigarette. He'd been chain-smoking since I woke. Obviously, rationing himself had not been an option.

He blew smoke out in a long exhale. "I'm a cop on holiday. What else have I got to do? Plus, with the state of your feet at the moment, you're about as useful as an ashtray on a motorbike."

I smiled. "True. I'll give Charlie a list of things to grab from the ambulance station, if he can get past Albert. I might also need some antibiotics."

Giallo studied the butt end left in his fingers and made a last attempt to suck the dregs from it, before grinding it into the stub-littered plate next to him. They looked like little tombstones in a miniature cemetery. "So, we're talking about ten days to wait and prepare before there's a chance of their return."

"About that. They said it's a two week round trip, and they left early on Friday."

"And Oz is the man to watch, but we can't afford to spook him."

"Right."

"Where's he live?"

"His place is on the outskirts of Gununa, but I'm guessing he might have some setup near Yuwah Point."

"Well, I better make a list, and I'll need a map. I haven't a clue where any of these places are."

"You'll be lucky to find a map. Probably be more useful if we had a laptop. I could then use Rob's satphone to access the internet."

"Got one?"

"Yes, but someone'll have to break into my donga to get it."

Giallo shot to his feet. "Hear that?"

I strained my ears. "A car?"

"He's made good time. That's my next pack of smokes."

"Better check it's Charlie. I'd hate for it to be anyone else. Remember, I'm a dead man."

Giallo nodded and strode out of the room. I heard the vehicle pull up outside and then voices, but they were too far away to discern. Soon after, the front door opened and the two of them came walking in.

"Hell, why you boys not got the aircon on? Surprised you ain't gone troppo in this heat, eh."

Giallo and I looked at each other, then back at Charlie. "You said you were getting fuel for the genny."

"That's for night time and as a backup. This place has a

shit-ton of solar panels." He flipped a switch to demonstrate, and the aircon stuttered into life.

We both swore in unison as Charlie boomed out a laugh. "I thought you were supposed to be a detective, eh, Gee?"

"You better have my smokes with you."

"Your bag's in the cab. Give me a hand off-loadin' and I'll cook us all a fry-up, while Jono here brings me up to speed, eh."

After they brought everything inside, they transferred me to a seat by the kitchen table. As Charlie threw various items into a large frying pan, I once again relayed my story.

But at the point I mentioned Oz, Charlie stopped cooking and turned to stare at me. "Oz?"

"Yes, he's their island contact. Why, what's up?"

"He was askin' me lots of questions, mainly about you, Gee."

"When?"

"Just before coming out here."

"What did you say?"

He looked to the ceiling, recalling his conversation. "He asked about the boat trip and I gave him some excuse about you trying to find the croc."

"Anything else?"

He sighed. "I might have said I thought the whole croc story was bullshit."

"Christ Charlie, d'you tell him I'm still alive?"

"No, nothin' like that. How was I supposed to know he was involved?"

Giallo tried to calm the situation. "Well, from now on, we all need to be a lot more careful. Is there any chance you were followed?"

"I don't..."

Everyone froze. Over the sizzling and spitting of the bacon rashers came the unmistakable sound of an approaching four-wheel drive.

28

CAUGHT

I was the first to react. Dropping to my knees, I scuttled on all fours to the bedroom, being as quiet as the wooden floor allowed. Once inside, I closed the door, but left a gap to see and hear what was going on.

The screen banged as Charlie went outside and Giallo lit up from his new pack of smokes. The car came to a halt, and I made my way over to the window, climbing on the bed, trying not to disturb the curtains. I peered above the windowsill and saw a white Nissan Patrol parked next to Charlie's dual cab. It wasn't Oz's ute.

Charlie was talking to a squat man who was wearing shorts and a loud Hawaiian shirt. He was waving his arms, but both of them were smiling, and I could just about make out their conversation.

"You came all the way out here to check I was all good?"

"Course. You're my favourite nephew." He laughed and gave Charlie a pat on the back. "Well, if truth be known, I was lookin' for an excuse to get away from your auntie for a few hours."

Charlie grinned and nodded. "That makes more sense. But I'd be grateful if you could keep it to yourself I'm here, eh. Police business an' all, y'know."

"No worries."

Charlie gestured towards the house. "You want to join us for some tucker?"

"Nah, I've already eaten. If you're all good, I'll be off. Beautiful day for a drive. In the peace and quiet. With no naggin'. All on me own. Might stop for a bit of fishin' on the way back."

He winked, and they shook hands. Then he got in his car and drove off with a wave and a cloud of dust.

I crawled into the kitchen, and Giallo watched as I pulled myself up onto a chair. "Did you hear any of that?"

"Yep."

"We're gonna have to sort your feet out."

"That's the next priority after some food."

Charlie walked back in. "OK, OK, don't give me any shit, he's the only one who knows I'm here, eh. It's his house, I had to ask, but I'm sure he can be trusted."

Giallo rubbed his chin. "Let's hope you're right. We haven't a clue if anyone else on the island's involved, so from now on, secrecy's essential and I guess the search for Jono's croc will have to be our cover."

Charlie nodded, then shrugged his shoulders. "So why are we hiding out and not just reporting this? All I know is that Oz is in with some sort of people-smugglin' gang."

"Well, you get back to cooking and I'll finish my story."

The acetate-like wings of a huge beetle fluttered to frustrate the force of gravity. The noisy creature had no right to be airborne, being large and without any aerodynamic shape. Nevertheless it flew, making an unerring bee-line towards the brilliant globe in its sights. Evolving millions of years before the advent of artificial bulbs caused constant confusion for its rudimentary brain. And as a result, it joined the rest of its insect cousins, buzzing around the floodlight aimed at the Gununa youth club basketball court.

"Three pointer comin' up."

The local teenager made a slight jump, and the ball flew from his grip, floating in a graceful arc before slamming through the hoop with a satisfying 'thock'.

"And the crowd goes wild."

He ran across the playing area, waving his hands high and trying to imitate the sound of roaring spectators as Charlie looked on. "Not bad, Dylan, but can you do that from the free-throw line?"

"Course I can, it's closer."

"Go on then. Ten bucks says you can't, eh."

The teenager frowned, but retrieved the ball and bounced it with each loping stride as he moved over to the top of the key. "You're on."

Taking up a shooter's stance, he bounced the ball while staring at the target.

"C'mon. You only get five seconds for a free throw. Five, four, three, two… Girls over there!"

The boy twisted his neck in the direction Charlie pointed as the ball left his hands. Once again it sailed through the air, but this time it rattled off the backboard, hitting the ring and bouncing over to the side.

"Guess you owe me a tenner, eh."

"That ain't fair, you distracted me!"

"You think the crowd'll stay quiet for your shot? You need to block out everything else. Total focus. Just you, the ball and the hoop, eh. Get that right and then the crowd will go wild."

"Double or quits?"

"Nah. I've gotta be off. You practise free throws for half an hour and I'll let you off the tenner. Work on your concentration, eh."

Charlie grinned at him and wandered off across the court towards the hospital. His undercover vigil was over. Albert had just left in one of the Troopies.

Reaching the building, a glance through the small square window in the side entrance near the ambulance bay revealed the coast was clear. He stepped through and went to the office, punching in the code on the keypad. There was a buzz, and he slipped inside, leaving the door ajar. Once in the room, he got out the shopping list Jono had made for medical supplies.

"Shit, with handwriting like this, he shoulda been a doctor."

But Albert's borderline OCD tendencies meant he stored everything in alphabetical order. So Charlie worked his way along the rows of boxes and collected the specified items, throwing each one into his back pack.

After rechecking the list, he zipped up his bag and turned to walk out, only to find Albert standing in the doorway, watching him.

"Jesus, you scared the shit out of me, Albert."

"What are you doing in my office, Charlie?"

"I came here to ask a favour, eh."

"Really?"

"Yep. It's about Jono. I wanted to help look for him, or at least search for the croc that's taken him. Do you have a problem with me borrowin' his boat?"

Albert took a few steps into the room and made an obvious, slow visual inspection. As he walked around his desk, he traced the edge with his hand and then slumped down onto his wheelie chair, staring at Charlie. After a long silence, Albert was the first to speak. "I don't care what you do with his stuff, I'm not his keeper. What does concern me is when you break into my office."

"Break in? The door was open."

"Charlie, I'm not Jono. I stick to protocols and follow guidelines. I keep the ambulances locked and I sure as hell lock my office door when I leave."

Charlie shrugged, and there was another long silence while they just stared at each other.

This time Charlie spoke first. "I'll swing by and pick up the boat tomorrow mornin' then. Catch ya later Albert."

He made a move to go, but the Station Officer stopped him in his tracks. "What's in the bag, Charlie?"

He turned back to Albert. "My footie boots, why?"

Albert sighed and shook his head. "Look, whatever arrangement you and Jono had in the past is over. He's gone, and he's unlikely to return. We're all shocked by what's happened and I know you two were close, so I'm prepared to turn a blind eye to the events here tonight. But from now on, there'll be no more helping yourself to medical supplies and I'll be changing the passcode for the office. Am I making myself clear?"

Charlie held his stare, then turned and walked out, calling back over his shoulder. "Don't know what you're talkin' about, Albert."

*

They had been bumping along unsealed tracks, turning at unmarked junctions and winding a path through monotonous, scrubby terrain for well over an hour when Charlie turned to

Giallo. "So, you sure you'll be able to find your way back to the house, eh?"

"I'm a detective. There aren't too many roads on this island. Plus, I plugged the location into my phone. Shouldn't be too difficult."

"Just take it easy when the trailer's attached. Some of these potholes could flip it."

"I intend to. I've had enough of your crazy driving."

"Hey, we could always swap and you sail the boat round, eh."

"Yeah right. There's no fear of that happening."

Charlie grinned, then pointed up ahead. "Here we are, back at Gununa. See that big white buildin'? That's the hospital. Jono's donga's in front of it, the one on the left."

As they drew nearer, the shrubs gave way to a flattened expanse, which Giallo realised was the bottom end of the runway.

"Better duck, Gee."

"Wha…?"

His response was lost in the roar of a twin-engine turbo-prop coming into land over the top of their cab.

"Jesus!"

Charlie boomed out a laugh. "You should see your face, eh. It's as if you ain't had a plane dive bomb you before. That must be an RFDS pickup."

"A what?"

"Royal Flying Doctor Service. Hopefully it means Albert's dealin' with a patient. That'll be one complication out the way. I thought he was going to do a citizen's arrest on me yester-day, eh."

"Doesn't your Police Liaison badge count for much?"

"Not if I'm caught stealin'. I'd lose me job. Anyways, this is Jono's place, and that's Albert's."

He pulled up outside a couple of lowset prefabricated buildings mounted on short stumps. They looked almost new, with security screens on all the windows, as well as solar panels and solar hot-water tanks on each roof. A large Poinciana sat between them, providing some shade, with its bright orange flowers scattered over a communal lawn scorched brown by the sun.

"D'you want to have a look around inside while I hook up the trailer? He's got an interesting wall in the back bedroom. That's also where you'll find his laptop."

"OK."

Giallo opened the cab and the mid-morning heat sapped his energy in an instant. He walked over to the short flight of steps and had a lit cigarette in his hand as he tried the front door.

It was unlocked, and he wandered inside, taking the time to observe each living space. There was a pile of dishes left in the sink and a few books strewn next to the sofa, but nothing looked disturbed. Nothing appeared out of place. He made his way to the back bedroom down a short corridor and hesitated for a second before turning the handle and pushing open the door. Fine lines of light crept between each slat of a closed blind masking the only window, and an air conditioner hummed a welcome. A screen saver waltzed an ever-changing pattern of lights around the monitor of an opened laptop, but most of the room was as dark and cold as a tomb. He flipped on a switch and the central ceiling lamp illuminated the sparse furnishings, the major focus of which was a complex collage covering one complete wall.

Giallo stared at it for a while before shaking his head. "Shit, Jono. You need to get yourself another girlfriend."

"Bit late for that, don't you think?"

"Jesus!" Giallo whirled around to find a short, fit-looking

man with leathery, tanned skin and close-cropped grey hair standing in the hallway. He was wearing a faded paramedic uniform and was staring at him with accusatory pale blue eyes.

The policeman recovered his composure. “I guess you must be Albert. I’m Detective Giallo, from Brisbane.”

He held out a hand, which Albert left hanging for a fraction too long before unfolding his arms and giving a curt handshake. “Why are you here? I’ve received no notification, nor explanation as to your presence on the island.”

“I’m not here in any official capacity. I’m actually on leave.”

Albert refolded his arms. “So… I’ll ask again, why are you here? I presume you haven’t got a search warrant, or permission to wander onto ambulance-service property.”

Giallo sighed and pointed to the wall. “That is why I’m here. I’ve been trying to track down the serial killer Jono unearthed last year. We’ve been working together on the investigation and I wanted to know if his recent disappearance was connected in any way.”

Albert cocked his head to one side. “You suggesting a croc might not have taken him?”

“It was something I was considering, but it doesn’t appear too promising. My intention was to take a few photos of this wall and borrow his laptop. See what I could find. Are you OK with that?”

Before he could answer, Charlie clattered his way into the house. “C’mon Gee, let’s get a move on. Don’t know when… Oh, g’day Albert. Thought you’d be dealin’ with the RFDS.”

Albert’s shoulders flexed as he tightened his folded arms. “And the plot thickens. Did you think I wouldn’t be here, Charlie? That was just some medical staff arriving for their rounds. No need for my services.”

He leant against the doorjamb and turned his head so he could see both of them. “Curious. Two people break into ambulance-service property on successive days and ask to 'borrow' Jono's stuff. Anything going on that I should know about?"

Giallo took a drag from his cigarette. "I didn't break in, the door was open."

Albert nodded towards Charlie. "Funny, that's exactly what your mate said yesterday."

Charlie smiled. "But didn't you say you weren't Jono's keeper, Albert?"

"That was yesterday. Now I'm not so sure."

The three of them stood looking at one another, the hum of the air-conditioning unit the only sound. Then Albert broke the deadlock. "You got any ID?"

Giallo pulled out his warrant card from his back pocket and handed it to Albert, who inspected the photograph, and then nodded his satisfaction. "I'll let you take the laptop now, but I want an official receipt for it by 5:00 PM today. I'll accept an email. Here's my address."

He presented Giallo with a business card. "Any further requests will be made upfront, by approaching me, not going behind my back. Am I making myself clear? You might think this is just an outback town, but I'm the Station Officer around here. Some professional courtesy would be appreciated. I can do without a rogue investigator roaming the island at the moment. Because of Jono's 'disappearance', I'm having to run the station, as well as cover his shifts until they send me a replacement. And that'll no doubt be a newly qualified graduate who needs babysitting, so I've got enough on my plate."

"Sorry. I had no intention of offending you."

"Well. I think I've made my point."

He nodded, spun on his heels and marched out of the house, his boots clumping on the wooden floors.

Giallo furrowed his brow, wondering how the man had crept up on him. He then took another drag on his cigarette and turned to Charlie. "Is he always such an officious bastard?"

Charlie grinned. "You caught him on a good day. I'm surprised he let you have the laptop without submitting signed documentation in triplicate, eh."

"Shit. I can't imagine him and Jono getting along."

He shrugged. "Hey, Jono's last station officer was a serial killer. I guess on that scale, Albert's a step up."

After finishing in the house, they drove round to the fuel station and filled up the ute and the marine tanks before making their way to the boat ramp. As they approached, Charlie slowed and pulled over. A small crowd had gathered at the jetty where a fishing boat was moored. On the back deck, suspended from a gantry, was the body of a large crocodile.

"You stay here, Gee. I'd better go find out what's happenin'."

Charlie left the car and walked over towards the gathering to the sound of raised voices. There was a man on the jetty, wearing a green cap, shorts and a cream-coloured shirt sporting badges from the Queensland Parks and Wildlife Service. He was arguing with Oz, who was standing on the deck of his boat.

"Look, mate, I had every right to kill it. I'm a single operator and when I was winchin' the cage, it began thrashin'. It threatened to capsize me, and the winch was failing. It took just one shot. I was humane."

The head of the croc bore testament to Oz's story, its left side being a mangled mess of torn tissue and bone. Rivulets of blood ran down its immense scaly body and the sun reflected off red droplets as they dripped from its gaping, downturned jaws.

The wildlife officer put his hands on his hips. "That's something we can discuss later, but you're not opening it up here."

"Why not? The ambo had no relatives on the island and it's gotta be the quickest way of knowin' if I've caught the right croc."

"Think about the effect on all these people if there's... evidence inside."

Oz addressed the crowd. "Anyone got a problem with this?"

There was a murmur of indifference, but the faces looked like those of onlookers at a hanging. Morbid fascination mixed with horrified excitement. Oz turned back to the wildlife officer and shrugged. "Can't hear any objections."

"It's inappropriate and against protocol."

Oz picked up a large filleting knife and walked towards the carcass. "Fuck protocol."

"You do and I'll see your licence is revoked."

He turned and waved the knife at the official. "Tell you what, how's about you accept my resignation."

With that, he reached up high and plunged the blade into the animal's neck, creating a split all the way down its belly with a single vertical stroke. Blood and entrails oozed out of the gaping rent in its tough skin.

"I order you to stop!"

The exasperated man spotted Charlie. "You there. You're with the police. Stop him. Stop him now."

Oz ignored him and reached inside to find the gizzard, splitting it open along with the stomach and spilling the contents onto the deck. Among the collection of stones, tissue and fragments of bone, was a black webbing belt, complete with a multitool and a stethoscope pouch.

All the commotion ceased and everyone stared at the mucus-covered garment. Oz broke the silence. “Guess we can call off the search.”

“That’ll be my decision, but you’re in a lot of trouble.”

Oz shrugged. “Like I give a shit. I don’t work for you no more.”

Charlie had walked up beside the Wildlife Officer, and Oz gave him a nod. “Charlie. Sorry for your loss. As I said before, it’s a fuck of a way to go.”

He grabbed a rag and wiped the blood from his hands. “Suppose everyone’ll have to return home now, including that city cop of yours.”

Charlie rubbed his nose. “Right. I guess so, eh. I’ll go tell him what you found.”

He strode off towards the waiting dual cab. Once there, he swung himself into the driver’s seat and without a word, slotted the transmission into drive and manoeuvred the car to head back the way they came.

Giallo looked at him. “What’s happened?”

“We need a slight change of plan. I’m going to launch the boat from Gee Wee Point and you can drive the trailer from there, eh.”

“Why?”

“Oz just made a show of finding Jono’s croc. It wasn’t the big one that I saw, y’know Punch, but now I’ve lost the reason for taking the boat and you’ll have to leave Mornington.”

29

MR GADGET

The three of us were sitting around the kitchen table, each nursing an ice-cold can of soft drink and dwelling on our own thoughts. My boat was now back on its trailer and hidden from view behind the house. At least I'd have a means of escape when the rains came, if I needed one.

Although it was mid-afternoon, the sun was still punishing the land, and the only place to be was in the air conditioning.

"Did you remember to send that email to Albert?"

Giallo nodded. "Called the office and got Melissa to sort it out. Last thing we need is Albert stirring up shit. Were you able to hook your laptop up to the internet?"

"Yep. Tethered it to the satphone, so I'm getting a great signal. Gotta hope Rob doesn't check his phone bill, though."

"A doctor who can afford a marlin boat spending time to read his bills? Seems unlikely."

Charlie decided to tackle the elephant in the room. "So. What we gonna do about you, Gee?"

He sighed. "I've an excuse to stay tonight, but any longer, and Oz'll get suspicious. He obviously wants me gone."

I took a mouthful of my drink and returned the can to the table, sliding it around the surface to make patterns with the condensation. "We could turn this to our advantage."

"How?"

"Well, I'm sure you could acquire some surveillance equipment in Brissie. If you fly there and pick up what we need, then all you've got to do is return to Mornington without being detected."

"And how d'you suggest that, Einstein? A plane's out of the question as there's only two runways that are easily observed, and as to a boat... I have to draw the line somewhere. It'll be a cold day in hell before I get back in one of those things."

"Perhaps we could use a large catapult and fire him from the mainland, eh?"

"Thanks for that Charlie. Surely there must be some way to smuggle him in?"

"Smuggle? Shit, why didn't I think of that sooner?" Charlie grabbed his phone and started searching through his contacts. "Gee, you got a pen? Here, write this number down. D'you reckon you could make it to Karumba?"

"Shouldn't be impossible. Why?"

"When you arrive there, you need to find this guy. I'm gonna call in a favour. He'll be able to get you here, under the radar, no doubt about it."

Giallo gave him a sceptical look. "And definitely no boat?"

Charlie held up his hand. "Scout's honour."

I laughed. "Since when have you been a scout, Charlie?"

Rain pelted off the tin roof and caused tiny explosions in the dirt around the house as the heavy droplets hit the ground. The noise was deafening, but I was treated to a pungent petrichor, that beautiful earthy smell that often accompanies a sudden downpour. I took in a deep breath to appreciate the aroma and not for the first time had to fight the urge to head back to Gununa to retrieve my coffee machine.

However, I was under house arrest. I couldn't go wandering outside and risk being seen. Even at a distance, a white guy around here would be noteworthy. Charlie had offered to bring some boot polish to blacken my face, but I knew he was taking the piss. This was going to be a waiting game, but the three days since Gee's departure had at least allowed my feet to begin healing. They were still tender and scarred, but when I had them bandaged I could walk on them, so long as I was careful.

Through the screen door I could see the rain accumulating in puddles and flowing down inclines. The rainy season would soon be on us, which would make any surveillance of Oz even more difficult, but at least we had my boat as an option. Hopefully, this would all be over before any serious cyclones kicked in.

A distant rumble of thunder gave me a fleeting flashback of the raft and how close I'd come to giving up. I shuddered and had to smile. A shrink could write a thesis on me and still have enough material left over for a lecture course. On a positive note, Amber seemed to have taken a back seat for a while, and I was getting the best sleep I'd had in months.

There was a buzz from the satphone, and I hobbled over to view the screen. It was a text message:

`No need to hide, only me`

I strained to listen for Charlie's ute, but could pick up nothing over the drumming rain. A few minutes later he pulled up outside with an enormous splash of mud and after a pause, came running to the house wearing his Akubra and a long Drizabone.

He burst in through the door, bringing a spray of water with him. "Jeez it's pissin' down, eh. Where'd that come from?"

"G'day Charlie, what's the news?"

He shook off his hat and coat as he removed them.

"Well, it's official."

"What is?"

"You've gone from missing to dead. They're holding a service for you on the island next Thursday and your ambulance lot'll run another the following week down in Brisbane."

"Great." I snorted a laugh. "Just think of all those managers who'll have to stand up and lie through their teeth. Guess that's business as usual for them. You going to the island one?"

"Course. Gotta pay me respects, eh. After all, I'm givin' the eulogy."

"Oh shit. How d'you land that?"

"Albert asked me. Apparently it was his responsibility, but I told him I thought 'good riddance' was far too short for a speech, eh."

"Fuck off."

"Funny, that was his other suggestion."

He ducked to avoid the ball of paper I threw at him. "So come on, other than that, what's been happening?"

At that moment the rain stopped as sudden as it started and I realised I'd been shouting.

Charlie looked up at the ceiling. "Ah, that'd be right. A few more minutes in the car and I woulda been dry."

"You were covered head to toe in waterproofs."

"Not the point. I'll go get the supplies I brought you in a

minute, but I just had to warn you that Gee should be back some time today."

"Today? Really?"

"Yep, you better tidy the place up."

"Yer right. What's the latest with Oz?"

"Nothin'."

"Nothing?"

"He's his grumpy, reclusive self, eh. It's not like I can observe him too closely, but if I didn't know better, I'd say you must be mistaken. I guess it's hard to believe anyone you know is a cold-blooded killer."

"Well, to be fair to Oz, as far as I'm aware he hasn't killed anyone yet. But he's just as guilty as the rest."

I stood and crept with obvious pain over to the fridge.

"D'you want me to do that?"

"No. I've got to start using my feet again. Wanna drink?"

"Sure."

Although Charlie had been back once before, it was good to have someone to talk to. I threw him a can. "So what've you been up to?"

"Not much, just my usual liaison stuff. Had a couple of things to organise for the youth club and footie training last night. Oh yes, Albert's got a temporary replacement for you. Arrived this mornin'."

"That was quick."

"You've been gone a week."

"Still. What's he like?"

"She. A pretty young blonde girl, looks all of twenty, eh. I was thinkin' of makin' a play for her, new blood 'n' all. Any chance you can stay dead so we can keep her?"

I grinned as I shook my head. "Don't get distracted Charlie. There'll be plenty of time for that sorta thing when we've caught the bad guys."

"Well, until Gee gets back we can't start any serious surveillance..."

His face broke into a beaming smile. "Hey, speak of the Devil."

"What?"

"Can't you hear that? You white boys have got crap ears, eh."

"Hear what?"

He raised his finger in the air and stared at me. "That."

I concentrated for a while, then shrugged.

"C'mon cripple, let's go meet 'im, eh. I'll show you what I mean."

He walked outside and down to the beach and I caught up with him in my own sweet time. It was like walking barefoot on gravel; every so often there'd be that inevitable sharp stone.

As I drew alongside him, he pointed out to the horizon. "There."

I squinted and made out a white dot travelling close to the water. "How the hell did you hear that in there?"

"Dunno. Any sound that's unnatural stands out, eh. Guess it's a blackfella thing."

"Right. It's either that or your big fuckin' ears."

He laughed and slapped me on the back. Then we watched as the speck grew bigger. "So, you never said why this guy owed you a favour."

Charlie gave me a smile and looked away. "Caught him trying to smuggle in booze to the island a few months after the pub closed. I shoulda turned him in. Problem was, it was a rellie of mine who was at the receivin' end."

He rubbed his chin. "Told the pilot if he took his cargo back and didn't return I'd let him go, eh."

I shrugged. "And he's flying in Gee just for that?"

He gave me a sideways glance and returned his focus to the

dot. "If I'd reported him he'd be up for a forty grand fine and would've lost his seaplane."

"Shit."

"Yep."

The dot had got larger and I could now make out floats hanging below the single prop plane. The drone of the engine changed in tone as it descended the short distance to the water's surface. Then there was a stream of white as it landed and taxied over towards us. The pilot manoeuvred his craft over to the beach and a side door opened. Seconds later, Gee clambered out onto one of the floats and vomited into the water.

Charlie and I were laughing when Gee looked up. "Scout's honour, my arse! A plane strapped to two canoes is still a fuckin' boat."

We helped offload Gee's bags and within minutes the engine was letting out a high-pitched whine and the seaplane left in a frothing wake. It was obvious the pilot had made the journey under duress and was not interested in small talk. He was off as soon as his debt was paid.

Gee sat on the sand, smoking a cigarette. He was wearing jeans, but they were baggier than before and he had a light cotton short-sleeved shirt.

I flopped down beside him to give my feet a rest. "You still don't look dressed for the tropics, Gee."

"I don't do shorts. Only my lady friends get to see my legs."

"Bet that's a treat for them."

He glanced at me, then went back to staring at the sea.

"How was your trip?"

"Long." He shook his head. "Don't know what it is about the sea. I've spent hours in different planes, with take off and turbulence. Not a flicker. But the instant I feel that water motion I'm yakin'."

"We all have our Achilles' heel, Gee."

He got up and dusted off the sand from his jeans. "Bet Achilles wouldn't have been so famous if he kept spewing every time he stepped on a boat. On the subject of heels, how're your feet?"

I stood on my bandages. "Not too bad. Getting there. C'mon, let's get in the aircon."

We made off towards the house and on the way, Gee picked up the last remaining bag Charlie had left behind. As we walked inside, Charlie threw us both a can. "Here, have somethin' to clear that taste from your mouth, eh."

Giallo caught his as he dumped the bag and cracked it open. "Thanks. What's been happening here since I left?"

"Nothin' much, eh. Things've been quiet, everythin's sorta gone back to normal."

I sat down. "Biggest news is Charlie's having to write my eulogy."

"That'll be short. Perhaps you can add a word from his killer. Do crocodiles burp?"

"Up yours."

Giallo took a drink from the can and joined me at the table. "Actually, your death's all over the Brisbane news. That reporter of yours has been pestering me for a comment."

Caught off guard, I tried to remain nonchalant. "I have a reporter?"

"Don't play coy, Jono, remember I'm the detective, and your reaction then spoke louder than any words. No one made a big deal about it last year, but I picked up on the reporting coincidence. Y'know, how the same woman was on the byline for all the supposed sightings of you in Carnarvon Gorge. And then she later released the whole story as an exclusive. What was her name? Oh that's right, Michelle Ludkowski."

The stare over his can of Coke was unwavering as he took a swig.

Charlie grinned at me. "I haven't heard this. Did you pervert the course of justice, Jono? Tut... tut... tut... Whatever happened to ambos being the most trusted profession, eh?"

I shrugged. "What d'you want me to say? I needed a diversion, and I used her. She was a previous patient of mine and I reckon she felt she owed me one."

I looked down at the floor before continuing. "I'm not proud of many of the things I did at that time. But what was I supposed to do? Roll over and be accused of something I didn't do?"

"You could have trusted in due process."

I stared back at him. "D'you think I'd be here now?"

He smiled. "What? Considered dead after being eaten by a crocodile on a tropical island?"

"Good point."

He lit up another cigarette and took a deep drag. "Look, let's say you passed one of my tests. I was just looking for an honest answer. We're about to get into some grey territory and I want all of us to be on the level."

He looked at me, then Charlie, and we both nodded in return.

He shrugged. "Anyway, they reckon there'll be a high turnout at the service in Brisbane. They weren't sure where to hold it, seeing as you're an atheist. I suggested having the wake at an Outback Jacks, y'know the restaurant with the big croc on the ceiling."

I laughed. "Now that would be funny. C'mon, Gee, stop

stalling and show us what gadgets you've brought. I was hoping we'd get a run down like Q does with Bond."

"Give me a break. I work for the Queensland Police Service, not MI fuckin' six."

He stood and hefted a bag onto the table, unzipping it. The first item he pulled out was a gun in a compact holster. "That's my service issue Glock 22. No one but me touches that. Understood?"

We nodded.

"I did acquire two tasers, so you each get one of them. They're pretty simple to use: point and shoot, like this, but you need to be near your target to stand a chance of hitting it."

"How near?"

"These are X26s so their maximum range is ten metres, but that's pushing it. Both probes have to hit the person's body and they spread out as they go, so five is more realistic for a beginner."

He took a drag from his cigarette. "In close quarters you can jam the contacts against your target, though that just hurts. It doesn't incapacitate. Of course, we don't want to use any weapons, right?"

"Right."

"As to comms, I've got three mobile phones to stay in touch, complete with tiny bluetooth earpieces for hands-free operation. Tap once to pickup and disconnect, double tap to mute the integrated microphone. The police digital radios won't work up here and the analogue ones are too easy to pick up on a scanner. The mobiles are all switched to silent and I suggest you do the same for your own, Charlie. Don't want that going off at an inopportune moment."

He nodded and pulled out his phone to change the settings.

"Now for surveillance; two pairs of normal binoculars and a night-vision pair."

"Cool."

"No, this little thing is the cool bit. It's not only a GPS tracker that draws its power from a car's fuse box, but it also transmits any sounds made nearby. This means we can listen in to conversations in Oz's cab and know where he is minute-by-minute. We can pick up the feed from a laptop or even the dedicated phone app."

I raised my eyebrows. "Shit, I'm impressed."

"I got hold of two, the other's for his boat, which should have him covered. There's just a slight drawback." Giallo turned to Charlie. "Someone needs to install them."

30

SCISSORS, PAPER, ROCK

Oz would sometimes leave his boat moored to the jetty overnight, so getting the tracker installed in that had been simple. Charlie stole down there at about 2:00AM and just plugged the gadget beneath the dashboard. But the fisherman's ute was proving to be another matter.

When at home, he always parked in the same spot beside his house. Charlie could've made another night-time sortie, but he remembered how the car door would make an awful creak. So he waited for Oz to go fishing.

There had been a couple of false alarms when Oz went to his boat and just pottered around, but today he'd motored off down the Appel Channel and Charlie watched as his vessel disappeared behind Denham Island.

He reached up and tapped his earpiece. "Is your tech working, Gee?"

"Yep. Can't hear much over the clatter of his inboard, but he's tracking down the channel at a steady speed. If you can't see him, you should be good to go."

"OK."

Charlie slotted his car into drive and rolled the rest of the way down the road to the parking area near the boat ramp. He pulled up next to Oz's ute and looked around. There were a couple of men fishing under the shelter at the end of the jetty, but they'd be hard-pressed to see him given the angle of the parked cars.

"In position, eh. Still good to go?"

"Roger that, Mother Hen. Stop cluckin' and get your arse into gear."

"Yours ain't the arse on the line here."

"It is if you're caught with my surveillance equipment."

Charlie made one last furtive scope of the area before slipping out between the cars. Pulling on the door handle of Oz's ute, he breathed a sigh of relief as the catch released. But its characteristic creak seemed to echo around the shoreline and renewed his anxiety. He ducked inside and set to work attaching the tracker.

It took him longer than expected to prise away the fuse box cover. There were so many smears and grimy marks on the plastic that he had to be careful not to disturb them. After that, the install was pretty straightforward, and he was replacing the cover when he heard a crunch on the gravel outside.

His body froze. He was lying across the front seats, with his feet out of the open door, and was clueless as to who was watching him.

"What you doin' Charlie?"

He sat up to find the teenager, Paul Johnson, leaning on the bonnet with a curious expression.

"Oh… Hi Paul. How can I help?"

"Just wonderin' what you're doin' in Oz's ute."

There was a hissed voice from the earpiece. "Think of something fast, Charlie. Looks like Oz was only doing a circuit of Denham. He'll be able to see your location within minutes."

Charlie climbed from the ute and shut the creaking door. "Er... Look, Paul. It's official police business. You've gotta promise me you won't breathe a word of this."

He smiled and held up both hands in surrender. "Mum's the word."

Charlie swung himself into his own car and fired up the engine, winding down the window as he closed the door.

The youngster gave him a disarming smile. "Course, you won't mind me checking this out with Miles, will you, Charlie?"

Charlie started reversing and leant his arm on the window frame. "What do you want, Paul?"

"Freedom from cleanin' ambulances and the right to see me girlfriend."

Charlie grinned and shook his head. "Done. But if you blab about this to anyone, you'll get the same punishment for six months, eh."

"Your secret's safe with me, mate."

He gave a wave as Charlie drove away, and less than a minute later, Oz's boat chugged into view.

I looked up from my laptop at the sound of Charlie pulling up outside. He'd called ahead on his approach and so there was no need for me to dive into the back room.

He burst in through the screen door in his usual larger-than-life way. "Sorry I'm late, needed to swing by my place before coming here. Had to change my underwear after that near miss with Paul."

I shook my head. "I must say, Charlie, you're not too good

at this undercover lark. You've attempted three covert ops and someone's rumbled you each time."

"I've no idea where Paul came from, eh, and Albert's like a fuckin' cat."

Giallo agreed. "I can attest to that. He appeared in your place without a sound and that was on wooden floorboards."

I shrugged. "Must be his military training. He never told me what he did in the service of his country. For all we know he could've been a spook."

"Anyways, what's with all this wood and chicken wire you had me bring over, eh? You thinkin' of raisin' some poultry so you can pelt the bad guys with eggs?"

"I'll get to that, d'you want to hear the plan we've been working on?"

Giallo walked over to the door and lit a cigarette, while Charlie sat down at the table opposite me. "I'm all ears, Jono."

I turned my laptop round so we could both see the screen. "OK, so this is the satellite image focused on the area around Yuwah Point. We're presuming they'll use the same location to ferry the refugees from the trawler to the plane, but we've got a fallback plan if they make a change. Anyway, as you know, there's only a single road leading to the beach. It's long, straight, remote and sheltered from much of the rain, being on the leeward side of Mornington. I'm guessing they chose there as the road can function as a landing strip."

Charlie nodded. "Seems logical."

"Now, our primary concern is the welfare of the refugees, so we can't start anything until all of them have made it to the island. The idea is to trap them on the land by a pincer movement, taking out the plane and the tinnie they use as a ferry at the same time."

"What about the trawler?"

"Well, if we do things quiet enough, the skipper should be

some distance off and, from what I witnessed, he just waits for the return of the tinnie. Once we have the refugees safe, we'll deal with him, but I'll discuss that later."

"OK. Go on."

I got up and limped over to the fridge. "Drinks?"

"Yep. Your feet any better, eh?"

"Yes thanks, I'm due another ibuprofen so they're playing up at the moment."

I sat down and cracked my can. "Back to the pincer movement. Again the assumption is that they'll attempt the transfer in the dark. They said as much to me with the plane needing to land at night. So, when we suspect things are about to happen, I'll take my boat around during daylight to this point here. It'll give me a chance to check they've moored the trawler in place."

Charlie rubbed his chin. "Won't they pick you up on radar?"

"Probably, but are they going to worry about every passing fisherman?"

"Depends if they see you stop near that headland, eh."

Giallo flicked some ash out the door before speaking. "Told you that was an issue, and it's not just because I don't like boats. I think this part of the plan needs work, it's too risky."

I thought for a moment, then shrugged. "OK, we bite the bullet and dump my boat on the beach today. It means if that's not the location, we've lost some flexibility. And after I drop it off, I'll have to walk to the road for a pickup."

"Are you up to it?"

"I think so. Now you've got me a good pair of boots I should be fine."

"Hmm... No, we can't risk you fuckin' up your feet, eh. Just tell me where to leave the boat and Gee can pick me up."

I had to concede his point. "OK."

"So, what about the plane?"

"Well, that's the bit you'll not like, Charlie."

He frowned and rolled his head to one side, but said nothing.

"Put simply, we crash your ute into it."

"What?"

"You don't have to write it off, just damage the plane enough to prevent them taking off. In fact, the less noise you make the better."

He didn't appear happy about the idea, but I pressed on. "So, you're in your car and I'll be in position on the coast to take out the tinnie, while Gee moves in on the bad guys. From what we know, there should be only two of them, Oz and the deckhand, trying to herd twenty hooded refugees."

Giallo waved his cigarette at me. "You know, it would be better to even those odds."

"Who d'you have in mind, Gee?"

"Can't we trust the island's cop?"

I thought about Miles and my interactions with him. Would a man involved in a people smuggling racket be walking his dog the night their entire operation was falling apart? I made a decision. "Yes. And what's more he's got, Bruno, a big German shepherd he can bring to the party."

Charlie nodded. "I agree, but there's no need to tell him until the last minute. He'll stress too much otherwise, eh."

"OK, so you deal with the plane and the pilot. We have zip ties to use as handcuffs. I cut off their retreat to the trawler, then Gee, Miles and Bruno control the rest. Two guns and a dog better, Gee?"

"I'm happier."

"So, on to catching the skipper. The idea's simple, Charlie and I drive out in their tinnie and taser him as he appears on deck."

Charlie rubbed his face and gave me a glum expression. "You want me to pull holes in the plan now?"

"Be my guest. It's a work in progress. I reckon we've got at least three days to find any weak points."

Giallo took a drag on his cigarette. "You sure they said the round trip was two weeks?"

"Yes, but I've also plotted the distance and checked the timing."

Charlie's brow was furrowed. "What about noise? Say we're too loud and the trawler takes off."

"We could chase it, but at that point, does it matter? We can call in the coastguard or even the navy. Only the skipper'll be left on the boat. They could sink it for all I care."

He nodded. "What if there's another refugee like that knife thrower?"

I'd considered this, but I thought it unlikely. "I think she was a one-off, but I guess it would be prudent to consider anyone without a hood to be hostile."

He took a swig from his can. "So what d'you need the chicken wire for, eh?"

"Ah, I'm glad you asked me that. We have to make your dual cab look like a rock."

"What?"

"There's a good chance that the plane's fitted with either a thermal or image-intensifying camera. Or both. So we have to be prepared. Anything spotted on approach from the air could cause them to abort and drown the refugees, so we have to be hidden as the plane arrives."

"Does that mean covering ourselves in alfoil?"

I smirked. "No, definitely not. I've been searching the internet for the best solution, and all that aluminium foil does is distract your enemy by causing them to fall about laughing. You'll light up like a beacon on both forms of night vision."

"Oh."

"What you have to do is hide beneath something camouflaged and stop your body heat from warming the covering, or escaping out from under it. Then you're invisible. If I take the canopy off my boat, I can leave it upside down on the beach and that'll give me the perfect hiding spot. But the car is a different issue. Although you, and Gee, along with Miles and Bruno, can sit inside it, the hot engine will stand out like dog's balls on a thermal imager. Also, the moon is likely to be up, so an image intensifier'll give the pilot an unrestricted view of the surroundings."

"So...?"

"We're going to build an insulated covering that'll make your car look like a big rock. The plan is to transport it there in pieces and hide off to the side of the road after Oz has driven down there."

His mouth opened, and he stared at me, then Giallo, then back to me. "You're actually serious, aren't you?"

31

SAILFISH

Charlie was sitting in the front pew, just before the small raised area that served as an altar. Mourners were still filing into the low-set church hall and there would soon be standing room only. He looked around and saw a real cross-section of the community, people who felt it necessary to pay their respects to an ambo who had been here less than a year. Charlie wondered whether it was the role Jono represented, or was his mate, the likeable rogue, really this appreciated?

He scanned the faces and nodded to several of his own relatives and friends as his mobile vibrated in his pocket. He tapped the tiny earpiece to accept the call.

"Hey, Charlie. What's the turnout like?"

Charlie leant forward and cupped his nose and mouth in his hands, as if he was praying. "No one here Jono, the place is deserted."

"Funny. Must be only you and Oz there, seeing as the tracker has his car outside."

"OK, so the hall's packed, but everyone's smilin'. I guess they're glad to see the back of you, eh."

"C'mon Charlie, I'm sure there won't be a dry eye left in the house after your eulogy."

"Happy or sad, I haven't had to speak in front of this many people since me primary school nativity."

"Really? What role d'you play, the donkey?"

"Very funny, I'll have you know I was one of the wise men."

He was stopped from responding to the laughter in his ear when he felt someone tap him on his shoulder. He looked up to find Albert standing over him with a curious expression. "Er, Charlie, I think everyone's here. Perhaps you could see if the ceremony can start?"

"Yes, right… sure Albert. Let's get the ball rollin', eh."

Charlie walked around and spoke to the relevant people before returning to his pew next to Albert. A short time later, a community Elder began proceedings and the murmur of muted voices fell silent. Eventually, it was Charlie's turn to speak, and he loped over to the lectern. Pulling out a piece of paper covered in handwritten notes, he looked out across the sea of faces.

Pausing, he cleared his throat. "First, I wish to add my thanks for everyone comin' here today. I didn't know Jono was so popular, eh."

There was a ripple of laughter. "Now what can I say about Jono. Like all of us, he has his faults…"

There was a hissed voice from his earpiece. "Past tense, Charlie, past tense!"

"Er, sorry… Had… Had his faults, but he made up for them with his many admirable qualities. In his work as the island's ambo, nothing was too much for him and he would always go the extra mile, eh."

It was a weird experience being present at my own funeral. It was like those tales of people looking down on their own bodies during surgery. I considered cutting the line, but opted to mute the microphone and took the earpiece out. As I placed it on the table, the dot on the computer screen caught my eye. It was moving. I turned up the volume to reveal the sound of Oz's ute clattering along a road.

His voice broke through the background noise. "You made it here quick. Any issues with this batch?"

There was a pause, after which he continued. "All's good here, too. Everyone bought the croc story. You won't believe it, but I'm just leavin' the smarmy fucker's funeral service. Yeah, I know. So, it's all on for tonight, then. Sweet, I'm headin' out there now."

His voice stopped, and the car stereo began blaring out some crooning country ballad. I turned down the volume and called out to Giallo. "D'you get that Gee?"

Giallo came into the kitchen, combing his hair with his fingers and yawning. "I think half the island heard that awful country music. Oz must only have the one CD. Surely nobody likes that crap."

I stared at him, and he stopped in his tracks. "What?"

"Didn't you hear what he said?"

"No."

"He was on the phone to the skipper. He confirmed the transfer's happening tonight. We're on."

"Shit. You better get word to Charlie because we need his car and he's gotta grab Miles and Bruno."

I continued staring at him.

"What?"

"Right now he's giving my eulogy."

"Well, it's not like he's doing anything important. He'll have to cut it short, he's got work to do."

I put the earpiece back in and unmuted the microphone. Charlie's voice filled my head.

"… There he was, standing on the jetty with the line in his hand. Torn between the duties of a paramedic and bringin' in a sailfish…"

"Charlie, you've gotta wrap it up."

"… Wha'? Er… But like the true professional he was, he turned his back on the fish of a lifetime, handed over the reel, and ran off to care for his next patient…"

"I mean now, Charlie. Oz is on his way to the site. It's all going down tonight."

"… Er…"

"Think of something. We need you."

"… Er…"

For a moment Charlie stood staring at the congregation, all eyes fixed on him, and an uncomfortable silence pervaded the hall. People started looking at one another, then back at Charlie. Suddenly, to everyone's astonishment, he buried his head in his big hands and began sobbing. Deep resonant convulsive gasps echoed around the room, and when he looked up, his face was a picture of dismay. "He entrusted that reel to me… and… and I let him down… I failed him!"

His shoulders shook, accompanied by a few more resounding sobs. "I'm sorry… I can't do this."

Putting his face back in his hands, he stepped off the dais and stumbled down the aisle, pushing his way out the door. Once outside, he strode over to his car, climbed in and drove off before the people who had followed him out got the chance to catch up and console him.

As he sped along the road, a rather stunned voice spoke in his ear. “Shit mate, I just meant for you to shorten your story.”

Charlie shook his head. “You coulda fuckin’ said that. Me mind went blank, eh. I had another page of notes. Didn’t know what to say.”

“Well, I bet the island’ll be talking about that for a while.”

“My blubbin’ll be forgotten soon enough.”

“Why’s that?”

“If all goes according to plan tonight, you can make your return from the dead t’morra, eh. They’ll be tellin’ that fuckin’ story for years.”

32

ULURU

Charlie had brought Miles up to speed on the trip out to the house. The police officer had been unable to attend the service and was completing paperwork at the station. It took little persuasion to convince him to join our venture, and he now stood beside us, holding Bruno's leash. When they arrived, the dog had leapt from the ute tray and almost bowled me over in his enthusiastic greeting.

"Hey, hey. Look who remembers you, Jono. Shit, it's good to see you, mate."

He came over and gave me a big hug. "So glad to find out you didn't end up as croc fodder."

I had to fight the feelings of guilt that welled up. "I'm just sorry I had to keep everyone in the dark."

He shrugged and patted me on the back. "People'll understand. And if they don't, fuck 'em. From what I hear, there's twenty lives at stake."

The four of us were now standing in a line, each holding a can of cold soft drink with the dog sitting next to Miles, bolt upright, his long tongue hanging from his mouth as he panted in the afternoon sun. We must have looked like a XXXX advert without the beer.

"So that's it, eh?"

"Yep."

"You sure it'll work?"

We were all staring at the mud-covered chicken wire and wooden frame Gee and I had built to cover the car. The inside was insulated with thermal blankets stolen from the hospital.

I rubbed my chin. "It only needs to look like a rock through night vision."

"Looks like a three-year-old's attempt to craft Uluru out of cardboard 'n' sticky tape, eh."

"Less of your whinging, we've got to get it loaded and out, so you're in position in the next couple of hours. And don't forget, I've gotta hike out to my boat from the drop-off point, so we'd better be going."

"Just one question."

"Sure, Miles, go ahead."

"If we're all sitting in the cab with doors closed, how does the last quarter of the rock get in place?"

"Yes, well... Er... How should I put this? One of you has to lie in the ute tray."

The three of them looked at each another, and Giallo was the first to speak. "As I've already told Jono, it can't be me. My back's dodgy."

Miles nodded. "Bruno can't be in the tray in case he barks, so I guess I'll have to be in the cab. I'm the only one who can look after him."

Charlie frowned. "Whoa. Hold on, this is my fuckin' car, eh. How come I get to lie on the hard metal? We could be there for hours."

"You just have to be in hiding when the plane flies over. With your hearing, that should give you about ten minutes to slot the last piece in place. Grab a sleeping bag from the house for something to lie on. And anyway, spare a thought for me. I'll be lying on the wet sand under my boat. You've got it easy, mate."

"Huh. I think Miles and Gee have got it easy, eh."

Taking care not to break them, we loaded the pieces of our rock onto the back of the ute and secured them down. After making a final check that all the equipment was stowed and ready, we bundled into the cab and set off for Yuwah Point. On the way, I flipped open the laptop and checked the blip's location. The intensity of the red dot throbbed, innocent as a strong radial pulse, but I knew it showed only where Oz had parked his car. He could be roaming the headland, and if he found my boat, we were screwed.

33

WINDMILL

It was approaching dusk when I was dropped off on the roadside to begin my walk. We'd been driving at a crawl for some time to reduce any chance of a dust plume revealing our approach. The others still had over a kilometre to go, but they decided to wait for darkness before taking up their position.

I wished them luck and started out through the dense scrub, carrying a few items in a small backpack. The sky blushed into gold as the sun set over the island, and my eyes had to adjust to the reduced light. I viewed the way ahead through the night-vision binoculars. Nothing stirred in the greenish glow.

My progress was slow as there were no paths and the terrain was rough. The moon was yet to rise, and even with regular night-vision checks, it was hard to see what was right in front of me. But at least my feet were holding out. Over the last few days, I'd been increasing my exercise and the new skin on my soles was hardening up.

I had to make my way down to the coast and then follow the land's edge to reach my boat. But before I could take up my hiding place, I needed to skirt the headland and scope the trawler. Walking on the beach would be relatively easy, but I still had to get there.

Thick stands of vegetation forced me to divert from my compass bearing and I'd lost count of how many cobwebs stuck to my face. But spiders weren't the problem; snakes were. I couldn't afford to disturb any sleeping under a bush, as Mornington was home to two species of venomous brown snake. I'd be lucky to survive a tangle with either of them.

The long hard slog in the dark reminded me of my walk from Lake Nuga Nuga last year, when I was on the run from the police. A few weeks ago, a memory such as that would have sent me down one of my mental wormholes, though tonight I brushed it off with a shrug. There were far more important things at play right now; but perhaps, like my feet, my mind was on the mend.

As I reached the sand, silvery light drenched the breaking waves, and it was easy to see where I was going. I glanced at my watch to discover it was still only 8:15 PM. I doubted the smugglers would try anything until after ten at the earliest. I set off along the strandline to hide my footprints and made much better headway, but it was past nine when I spotted the upturned hull of my boat. Looking at the shape, I realised something was wrong.

I stopped and used the binoculars to focus on the lower edge. "Shit. Just my fucking luck."

I pulled out my phone and dialled the car.

"Wassup Jono? You got eyes on the trawler already?"

"No, Charlie. There's a slight issue with my hiding place. What's the safest way to get a croc to piss off? Looks like Punch is lying right next to my boat."

There was a pause and I could tell from the tone of his

voice when he spoke he was stifling a laugh. "You not got a rollin' pin in that bag?"

"I've got a taser, which I'll use on your arse if you don't take this seriously."

"Calm down, Jono. Even the monster ones'll go back in the water, you just need to annoy it enough. Should be easy for you, eh. Try prodding it with a big stick."

"Right. A big stick?"

"Yer, but be ready to run, eh."

"Great. Glad I had a croc expert on hand to advise me."

I hung up and walked closer to my dilemma, looking for any decent-sized driftwood I could use. I spotted some further up the beach and went over to retrieve a piece. Having a two-metre club bolstered my confidence, but any bravado I'd accumulated dissipated when I saw the croc at close quarters. Punch was over five metres long — bigger than my tinnie. He eyed my advance with the disinterest you might reserve for a solitary ant approaching your sun lounger.

I held the branch out at arm's length and crept ever closer to the massive animal. The moonlight traced each edge of the knobbly scutes covering its body, and the armour-plated skin of its neck and belly sagged outwards under its own weight. Punch was lying up against my boat with his legs splayed out beside him, like some overweight mediaeval knight had just given up doing press-ups. Surely a croc this size couldn't be that quick on land. The thought spurred me on, and I called to it in a low voice. "Go on, you overgrown lizard, bugger off back to the water. This is my boat."

Nothing. I stretched closer and tapped his snout with the tip of my branch. His jaws opened like a blossoming flower and he let out an ominous hissing sound. Despite the dim light, I now had an unobstructed view of his impressive dentition, and my resolve was waning.

I took a deep breath. "OK. Charlie reckons I've just got to annoy you enough."

I landed another tap on his jaws and received a further hiss.

"Oh shit, here goes."

I belted his snout with the wood, which shattered into pieces. This time there was no hiss. Punch launched his immense body towards me, using his tail to add propulsion and his powerful jaws slammed shut just where my head had been a fraction of a second before.

In contrast, I had scrambled backwards, flailing my arms and legs like a windmill in a tornado, kicking up sand in my hasty retreat. And now, without even a glance behind me, or a thought about my damaged feet, I was sprinting full pelt along the strandline. Punch was an issue I'd have to deal with later.

34

VOLTS

I crept over the rocky headland, under cover of some low-lying bushes, and lay on the ground to observe the expanse of the bay. Moonlight was illuminating the scene, and the trawler was easy to see, ominous in its innocence, moored in the lee of Sydney Island.

I retrieved the binoculars, magnifying my view of the boat, and was surprised to discover the rig at the surface. As I watched, my phone vibrated and I tapped the earpiece. "Hey Charlie, looks like they'll be moving them soon, they've raised the shipping container."

"I hope you solved your croc problem, 'cos I can hear the plane, eh."

"Shit, I've just made it to the headland."

"Well, you better run, brutha. You gotta hide that heat of yours, eh."

Cutting the call, I crawled back from my vantage point, and, as I dropped from the trawler's line of sight, began sprinting along the beach. The distant sound of the aeroplane was audible over my laboured breathing as the shape of the upturned boat appeared in front of me. There was no sign of the croc, so I launched myself into a baseball-style slide and shot under the gap between hull and sand, clattering against the opposite side. To my horror, my arrival elicited a low grunting growl from outside. Punch had returned to his sleeping spot.

Every one of my muscles tensed, even my chest stopped breathing. The sound of the plane passing overhead was a mere distraction compared to the wait for what the croc would do next. His claws scraped on the metal and sand seeped under the edge as he raised himself up onto his short, squat legs. He was on the move, but which way? Back to the water? If he came round to the upturned side, I'd be trapped like the soft gooey centre of a fancy chocolate.

Each of his scales sounded like a cheese grater as his powerful tail dragged along the boat. Shit. He was walking up the beach. I cowered in the corner, as far away from the opening as possible, trying not to move. In the dim light, all I could think of was the image of those jaws snapping in my direction. Then my phone vibrated.

I tapped the earpiece and managed a whisper. "Not a good time."

"Guess you must've got to your hiding place 'cos the plane's landed. You should be safe to come out. We need your eyes on the operation, eh."

"Yeah, well, I'm busy. Y'know my croc issue? He never left. He's now cornered me under my boat."

"Dunna worry, Jono. Crocs don't hunt on land."

"Don't think this one's read the rule book."

As I was speaking, I'd reached into my bag and my hand curled around the handle of the taser. The probes wouldn't pierce his flesh, but I could still give him a jolt with the contacts. If he came close enough.

Suddenly Punch's snout thrust into the gap and swiped back and forth, scattering sand and blowing some in my face as he breathed hard through his nostrils. Before I was able to react, the jaws disappeared, and all I could hear was the thudding of my heart.

"You still there, Jono?"

I didn't dare speak. I was straining to listen for movement outside over the deafening pulse in my ears.

"Jono?"

Not a sound.

"Jono?"

Nothing

"Jono? You OK? I can hear you breathing."

From the continued silence, I reckoned it was safe to respond. "I think he's gone."

But I should've known better than to tempt fate. A moment later, his snout reappeared and in a single violent action, the enormous animal threw back his head and flipped the whole boat off me. I was left lying foetal on the sand, exposed beneath a moonlit sky in all my vulnerability.

For a second, the two of us just stared at one another. Then the croc lunged, jaws open, teeth bared. With all my strength, I jammed the taser between his nostrils and pulled the trigger. The contacts fizzed as they delivered a drive stun of fifty thousand volts into the sensitive part of Punch's nose. The reptile recoiled with a surprised, yelping bark and shook his head, before whipping around and galloping off down the beach.

Charlie's voice came through my earpiece. "What the fuck was that?"

My heart was still thudding, and I was lying in the same position on the sand, my arm outstretched holding the taser. "That, my friend, was the sound of a croc being tasered. Sure as hell beats your rolling pin."

"He must've liked you, eh."

I took a deep breath and sat up. "Where are you now? Have you guys moved?"

"No. We've cleared Uluru Two from the car, but we're waiting for your go ahead."

"Give me a couple of minutes. I'll get back to the headland."

I stood and brushed the sand off my clothes while admiring the taser. Gee was wrong. This gadget was by far the coolest thing he'd brought. I threw it in my bag and ran to the look-out, crawling under the bush before contacting Charlie.

"I'm counting ten hooded people kneeling in a group just inside the tree line and the tinnie is returning to the trawler. Assuming they're running with twenty customers again, they'll have to complete two more trips. I reckon Gee and Miles have at least thirty minutes to move into position. As to bad guys, there's the one in the tinnie, I'm guessing Bruce, and Oz is on the island with the refugees. I can't make out anyone on the trawler, but the pilot's staying with his plane that's about three hundred metres up the road from Oz."

"What sorta plane is it?"

I turned the binoculars to the aircraft. "I'm not too good with plane IDs, but it's a fat-bodied cargo type, about ten metres long with a single engine. All you need to do is clatter into the front of it and bend the prop. Then they'll be trapped here. I'm guessing there isn't anywhere to turn it around, so they must've landed coming in from the sea, which means they intend to take off towards you. Looks like Oz placed small lights along the road to guide it in."

"Right, keep us posted, eh."

"Sure, I've got nothing else to do for the next half hour."

35

CHAOS

Matt chewed on his cigar as he watched Bruce guide the last customer into the tinnie. "Keep on your toes. I won't be happy until we're steaming the fuck outta here. Think it's the moonlight that's spookin' me. Don't like everythin' bein' so fuckin' visible."

"I hear ya. I'm not gonna hang round for a chat. Chuck me the spare fuel tank and I'll be on my way. I think I'm gettin' low."

Matt grabbed a red plastic jerrycan from its stowage on the deck and handed it to Bruce. "Here, this one feels half full, but if you run out, you'll have plenty to get back." As Bruce clicked the outboard into gear, he threw the painter in the bow. "Go on, the sooner you dump this batch, the sooner we can fuck off."

Bruce twisted the throttle and touched the peak of his oily cap as he turned the boat to land. Unlike the last time, there was no need for Oz to leave his headlights on. It was bright enough to see the gap between the trees, and he opened up the engine once he was pointing at his mark.

He had to agree with Matt. This all felt too exposed. At least the next delivery would be during a new moon, but the weather was only going to get worse. Next time it was likely to be pissing down and fuck knows what the sea journey would be like.

A small wave clipped the side of the boat and splashed his face with spray. He licked the drops from his lips, enjoying the salty taste, and studied the five figures, hooded and huddled together. This was as near as he got to them, and their closeness created mixed emotions. In reality, the trips were like any other trawling stint, but the cargo was far more lucrative than prawns had been for years. These fuckers were his ticket to the life he always wanted. It's just he hated goddam immigrants, and it was him bringing more of them over here.

After a while, the waves breaking on the beach interrupted his thoughts, and he focused on getting the boat ashore in the semi-darkness. Once the keel was dug in the sand, he cut and lifted the engine and jumped overboard into the knee-deep water. The splash was met by a loud scream from the land.

He spun towards the sound, hand reaching to his waist, eyes scanning the dark scrub. But then he saw a bird running along the shore and realised it was only the cry of a stone curlew. He snorted a laugh and spat in its direction. He'd been told spitting was a tradition to ward off the death associated with the bird, and although he didn't believe that Abo crap, it was better safe than sorry. Either way, he could see his hand shaking in the moonlight before he gripped one of the hooded men by the shoulder.

"Right, out ya get." His instruction caused another man to stand. "You! Sit the fuck down now! Don't move until I grab your fuckin' arm."

When all five were kneeling on the beach, he pulled the boat up a few metres and dumped the anchor on the strandline. He had no intention of staying, but the process was automatic for a seasoned crewman.

"Right, get up and hold the person in front of you."

One refugee remained on his knees and Bruce dragged him to his feet, yanking his hand so he gripped the belt of the man next to him. "No speaky Engrish? Jesus, you're gonna do well."

He then grabbed the upper arm of the lead man and guided them over the sand, up to the larger group of refugees.

Oz nodded to him as he arrived. "Took your time. C'mon, let's go. I'm sick of standin' round here with my finger up my butt. Not sure why I couldn't start loadin' 'em."

Bruce shrugged. "Cos we're stickin' to the plan. The fuckin' plane wasn't supposed to be here until now."

They soon had the entire group on their feet, stumbling along the road with Oz leading the way, while Bruce bullied any stragglers. As they drew near the plane, the pilot leant out the side door and beckoned them to hurry.

Bruce shook his head. "Don't know what he's complainin' about. He's the one who arrived too fuckin' early."

Oz grinned. "Bloody pilots, think they're God's gift. They're just glorified taxi drivers. Bet he's got a tiny cock."

They were still laughing when they heard an approaching engine speeding their way. With his arm raised, the pilot turned to look, then leapt away from his plane as Charlie's dual-cab ute hurtled out of the night. A short distance before impact, the car hit a pothole and went airborne, smashing into the aircraft head on and glancing upwards. The plane's nose collapsed as the undercarriage buckled, and the ute ploughed through the cockpit, stopping with a thud of grinding metal when the bull bar met the wing's superstructure.

The pilot jumped up and stood aghast, staring at the destruction of his plane, then strode over to wreckage, reaching up to throw open the driver's door. "Are you fucking mad, you f… f… f… f… f…"

His expletive was drawn out for about five seconds as his body tensed like a board and his limbs fidgeted before he collapsed to the floor, hitting his head on a rock that knocked him unconscious.

Oz stared in disbelief. "What the fuck?"

Just then, two figures emerged from the undergrowth, one restraining a large growling dog and the other levelling his gun at Oz's chest. "Police! Nobody move! Keep your hands where I can see them."

Although the smugglers froze, the command caused panic among the hooded refugees. Several screamed, some dropped to the ground, and others started running, but they didn't get far as they bumped into one another, or tripped on the uneven road.

In the chaos, Bruce grabbed the nearest person in a headlock. Holding the unfortunate man's body in front of him like a shield, he whipped out a silenced handgun and pushed the suppressor against his victim's temple. "Fuck you! Keep that mutt on its leash, or I'll blow this cunt's brains out."

36

YOU

I gave the others a heads-up that the refugees were on the move and broke cover, running along the beach to get to their tinnie. The sand glowed in the moonlight, and I hoped the skipper wasn't watching the shoreline from the trawler.

As I reached the boat, I heard the crump of metal as Charlie hit the plane and tapped my earpiece to check he was OK. "Jesus, Charlie, sounds like you bulldozed it. What happened to just bending the prop?"

"Hey, it was dark with no headlights. I misjudged the distance, then hit a bump. Got the job done though, eh."

"You never do anything by halves, do you?"

"Hold on, here comes the pilot."

There was another voice in the background, then a crackle of static. "Wow. These tasers work well, eh. Pilot's down... and out. Oh fuck."

I'd disabled the outboard engine by removing the deadman clip from next to the throttle. "What's up?"

"Christ, everything's gone to shit. One of the bastards grabbed a hostage. Where are you?"

"By the boat."

"We could do with you here, now. Stealth mode, eh."

I swore under my breath and cut the call, creeping up the beach with my taser held low. So many times I'd been in dodgy situations, asking for police backup, but this was the first time I was the one going in armed. I wasn't sure which I preferred. Keeping to the shadows, I made my way adjacent to the road and could soon hear Bruce shouting orders.

"Throw your guns in the bushes and go tie that fuckin' dog up to a tree, before I shoot it."

Gee and Miles did as he demanded.

"Now, whoever's in that ute, get out slow and join the rest of these fuckers on the ground. That goes the same for you two cops. No quick movements, stay face down with your hands on the back of your heads."

All the refugees were already lying on the dusty road, apart from the one who was still gripped in a stranglehold. I had a good view of him now and was struck by the irony of the scene. How many of these people had fled their own country to avoid persecution and here they were, within the first hour of being on Australian soil, cowering in hoods while a deranged redneck threatened to kill them.

Bruce continued calling the shots. "Right, Oz. Go check the pilot."

Oz walked over to his slumped body. "He's out cold. Pissed himself as well."

"Shit. Search these bastards and take any phones off them, then grab yourself a hostage and come over here."

Oz shook his head. "Sorry, mate. You're on your own. Let's face it, the game's up. You ain't gonna make a getaway in a fuckin' trawler."

"I'll give it a damn good try. I'm figurin' they won't do anythin' with hostages on board. And what's more, where's the fuckin' SWAT team? I reckon it was just these three cockheads tryin' to be heroes."

"Cockheads or not, they know who I am and I'm too old for a life on the run."

"You sure?"

"Yep."

"Suit yourself. Been a pleasure workin' with you, Oz."

Bruce took the pistol from his hostage's head and fired two shots at the fisherman's chest. The muted sound from the silencer was like a couple of volleys from a paintball gun, but the dark stain that spread across Oz's shirt was no dye. He let out a gasp and fell to the floor, eyes wide and glazed.

"Right. Guess now you all know I'm not fuckin' about."

He waved to Charlie. "Hey you, coon. Collect up the phones, or I'll have to shoot the lot of you. The rest stay on the ground and don't look up."

I was almost in taser range when a dry branch broke under my weight, letting out a loud crack. Bruce whirled around and pointed the gun in my direction.

"Ha, so there's four cockheads. That's why you gave up so fuckin' easy. Come out of the shadows, you little shit."

I held up my hands and walked out into the silvery glow of the moonlight.

Bruce's mouth fell open. "You… It can't be. You're fuckin' dead. I saw you die."

He was waving the gun at me and released his grip on the hostage, who dropped to his knees, coughing and gasping for breath.

"The boat, it…"

As I watched his confused expression, his head ruptured in a cloud of gore. Blood, brain matter, and particles of bone sprayed out in a plume, and I felt the liquid pepper my face and clothes. Then his almost headless corpse stood for a moment, before collapsing onto the terrified man at his feet.

I blinked, finding it hard to comprehend what I'd just witnessed. Then I dropped to the ground. "Sniper! Everyone stay down."

Pulse racing, I scuttled over to where Gee and Miles were lying.

Gee was scanning the area. "What the fuck just happened?"

"I was hoping you could tell to me. D'you forget to mention you'd organised the cavalry?"

"I've got a hotline for the Feds, but I'm yet to ring it. This isn't me."

I called over to Charlie. "You have any ideas?"

"Haven't a clue, Jono. Could it be the skipper? He might've missed, eh?

"Not unless he's left the boat. The shot came from inland."

"Hey, guys, there's a car coming, eh."

"Is there?"

I looked at Gee and Miles, who both shrugged.

"Got a plan Gee?"

"Stay low. Cable tie the hands of the pilot and spread out into the undergrowth. Hide until we can determine if they're friendly."

"Right."

A couple of minutes later, we could all hear the approaching truck and I recognised the engine tone. "Well, I'll be fucked. I think I know who our saviour is."

I stood up and walked out from the bushes as the marked-up Troopie pulled up in front of the wreckage of the plane. Although the headlights were off, I could still read the word 'Ambulance' printed across the bonnet.

Albert stepped out of the cab and swung a rifle onto his

back. “G’day Jono, why weren’t you at this morning’s meeting?”

I shook my head and my face broke into a wide grin. “Had something better to do, Albert.”

Walking over to him, I gave him a big hug, lifting his stiff body off the ground. “You know, I never thought I’d say this, but it’s bloody good to see you.”

He squirmed to get away. “Put me down, you bastard. You’re getting claret on my uniform.”

I released him and stepped back, wiping the blood from my face. “It’s all from your handiwork.”

He shrugged. “It was the first opportunity I had for a clear shot and I took it. Pity I couldn’t save Oz. Looked like that guy had you all on the ropes.”

“Damn glad you’re good with that rifle. I take back all the shit I’ve given you about going pig hunting. Anyway, how d’you know we were here?”

Gee and Charlie had joined us while Miles had gone to untie Bruno.

“Things weren’t adding up about your disappearance and so I did my own detective work.” The corner of his mouth flickered. “Crocs have got more taste than to eat a smart-arse like you. And Charlie here might be a good tracker, but he never looks behind him.”

He nodded at the plane wreck. “Nice bit of parking.”

Charlie grinned. “Reckon I’ve blown my no claims.” Then his black forehead crinkled, and he turned to where the pilot was lying face down. He gave the man’s shoulder a kick, and the pilot rolled over. “Hey… Wha…?”

“Wake up. How come your thermal camera didn’t detect him and his Troopie, eh?”

The pilot gave Charlie a blank look. “What thermal camera?”

Everyone stared at me, and all I managed was a sheepish grin. "Hey, I only said it was a possibility."

Gee glared at me. "You had me making a mud model of Uluru for two fucking days."

Charlie started laughing and Albert just looked confused.

"At least you didn't have to taser Punch."

Gee's mouth dropped open, then he regained his composure. "I'm not even going there. No matter what that's all about, I think we've got some unfinished business. If you're still insistent on nabbing the skipper, you'd better be on your way."

I shrugged. "I don't want him to escape. He's our only link to the real boss of the operation. Besides, he's made things personal."

"Well, there's no point me joining you on the boat, and I need Miles here to handle Bruno. He might be useful if we have any runaways. Are you still up for this, Charlie?"

"Never backed away from a fight yet, eh."

"Right, the two of you mad bastards better get going. You might outnumber the captain two to one, but I'm calling in the Feds now. If there's any problem, back off and let them deal with him, OK?"

"Will do, Gee."

I turned to Albert. "You think you'd be able to offer any cover from the shore?"

"Not with this pig rifle. That's at least two K's. I'd need my Special Forces Barrett M82 for a shot like that. If I used this, I'm just as likely to hit one of you two."

For a moment, words failed me, but then I found my voice. "Albert. There's a whole side of you I know nothing about."

He shrugged. "You never asked."

I'd worked with this man for nine months and never got past his officious facade. Perhaps that was part of my problem.

Perhaps I was too quick to judge people without really getting to know them. Was it my ambo training, or did it hark back to the loss of my brother? Had my subconscious always feared losing someone again? No wonder Amber's murder had screwed with my head so much.

I nodded to him. "I will, Albert, but not now. C'mon Charlie, let's go."

As we walked away, Gee began organising things. "OK, Miles, best get the hoods off these folk, then group and count them."

I stopped at Bruce's body and knelt down to pick up his cap, shaking some tissue from the brim. "Here Charlie, give me a hand to remove his shirt. I've at least got to look a bit like him."

His face grimaced at the sight. "I guess you've seen worse shit than this, eh Jono?"

I glanced at the gaping hole in the front of his head and in a millisecond my mind flashed through a multitude of old trauma images, ending with Amber. Flashbacks were a consequence of my role and when they were people you knew they were harder to shake. But the rest? Like most paramedics, I could somehow suspend empathy and assign the view of some awful reality to just another job.

Once again, I shrugged my shoulders. "Yes. Don't think about it, mate, just get on and do. Make sure you talk about it afterwards, though, then you'll be OK. It's why ambos always tell their stories, it's part of our coping mechanism."

He started pulling at the shirt. "Christ, I couldn't do your job, eh. What we gonna do about all the blood?"

"I'll give it a rinse in the sea before we head out."

After replacing the deadman clip on the outboard, we were soon underway with Charlie lying under a tarp towards the bow of the boat. The trawler lay offshore, looking no different from any other moored vessel sitting at anchor, but the knowledge of who was on board made the peaceful scene appear like a set from a horror movie. A drop of salt water fell from the peak of Bruce's greasy cap and I pulled it down lower over my face.

After a while, I raised my voice just loud enough for Charlie to hear over the outboard. "About a kilometre to go. Still got a chance to back out, mate."

"No way, Jono. This is a better buzz than reelin' in that sailfish, eh."

"Well, let's make sure this bastard doesn't get away."

"Not this time. No worries."

We fell silent, and I had to admit he was right. My heart was thumping, mouth dry, teeth clenched, muscles tensed. The anticipation was intoxicating.

As we approached the fishing boat, I saw a figure standing at the gunwale and eased off on the throttle, dropping the revs.

"What took y'so long?"

Hoping the noise of the engine would mask my voice, I called back in my best Bruce impersonation. "Wheel of the fuckin' plane got stuck. Had to free it."

I clicked the shift lever into neutral and we coasted to the side.

"Well, move ya fuckin' arse, Bruce, or the skipper'll rip yer a new one."

Before the relevance of his warning sunk in, Charlie leapt out from under the tarp and fired his taser. The barbs hit the startled man in the chest, who forced out a stifled cry. His body went stiff and collapsed back on the deck with a heavy thud.

Everything then moved in slow motion.

Charlie turned to me grinning as one of the bridge doors flew open. Light spilled out and the skipper burst onto the landing, brandishing a hand gun. As he took aim, I managed to yell, "Get down, Charlie!"

Realising my taser was out of range, I grabbed the spare fuel tank by my feet and hurled it towards the skipper. I heard a blast as the bullet punctured the flying jerrycan, spraying fuel across the trawler's deck. Despite my efforts, the projectile continued on its trajectory and slammed into Charlie, flinging him overboard. For the second time in less than an hour, I had someone else's blood splash on my face.

My heart froze and all I could do was scream a single word. "Noooo!"

I scrambled to reach him, but the skipper's voice stopped me in my tracks. "Don't you fuckin' move."

Keeping still, I scanned the inky black water, looking for any movement, any bubbles, but realised I'd be no use to Charlie if I shared his fate. The deck lights flicked on and I could hear the skipper walking down the stairs. "Turn around you mother fucker. I don't like shooting people in the back, unless I have to."

I stood, ripping my eyes away from my desperate search, and turned towards him. Like Bruce, his mouth fell open when he saw who I was. "You! The fuckin' Ambulance Man? I killed you... Twice." He shook his head and wiped the spilled gasoline from his face. "You're like a fuckin' cockroach. This time I ain't gonna miss. I reckon third time lucky sounds about right."

He aimed the gun at my chest, but a calm had settled over

me. "What? You're going to shoot an unarmed man in cold blood. All I have is this taser."

I presented it to him, pointing the barrel to his side, and tapped the trigger. The barbs flew out and off in the direction of the trawler stairs.

The skipper laughed. "You fuckin' loser, ya missed. I'm gonna enjoy this."

I nodded to his left and echoed the words Amber used in one of my dreams as I squeezed down hard on the trigger. "You sure I missed?"

The barbs' contact with the metal stairs created a shower of sparks, and as the skipper turned to look, a fireball flashed towards him and engulfed his body. Staggering backwards, he tripped over his crewmate who was attempting to get up and they both fell in a sprawling heap among the flames dancing around the deck. Their screams pierced the night's air, as I leapt to the side of the tinnie and grabbed a flashlight from my pocket. Waving the beam underwater, I hoped to make out a dull shape, anything to guide my dive, but all that greeted me were a million shining specs of plankton. A myriad watery stars glowing back at me. Surely he couldn't have sunk that far? Surely it was too soon for his solar system to be snuffed out?

"No!"

I scrambled over to the other side, but was amazed to see a black hand clutching the edge and a set of white teeth gleaming in the flashlight. "Hey, Jono. Any chance you can stop fuckin' around with that torch and pull me up?"

I laughed and hauled him into the boat. I couldn't believe he'd survived. "Christ, am I glad to see you. I thought I'd lost you, mate."

He grinned. "Y'need more than one bullet to take down a blackfella, eh."

There was a neat hole in his shoulder and blood was oozing out, soaking his T-shirt and dribbling down his chest.

"After he shot me, I swam under the tinnie and hung on the opposite side, eh. Reckoned my best bet was to stay there and rock the boat if he took aim at you. Fuck this hurts. Sorry I wasn't much good to you, eh."

I ripped his top off and bundled up the material into a pad, pushing it against the wound. "You have no idea how good you've been for me, Charlie. Here, keep pressure on it with this. I know where there's an ambulance."

"Just make sure it's you who treats me, not Albert, eh."

I smiled at him. "No worries, mate."

As I motored away, there was an explosion from behind us and I turned to see the trawler ablaze. Even from this distance, I could feel the heat from the fishing vessel, which was burning within such an inferno it was lighting the night's sky like a mistimed sunset. I shook my head and looked back to the shore. A viking funeral was more than that fucker deserved.

37

EPILOGUE

Scotty pressed the remote for his car and the indicators of a bright red Ford Falcon flashed in response.

"What, no Camaro?"

He grinned. "C'mon boss. You know she only comes out on special occasions."

"Right. And my return from the dead ain't special enough?"

"Course it is, but you've got me driving into a shitty area of town." He shrugged. "You gotta admit that's too risky for her."

I laughed. "OK, I'll let you off."

I threw my bag into the open boot and climbed into the passenger seat. It was good to be back in Brisbane. The hustle and bustle of the airport, the milling people, the smell of coffee in the terminal, and the cool of the night breeze. I'd missed the place.

But this was just a flying visit. The powers that be had sanctioned my official return to the city in three months' time. Today I was here to take someone home.

Scotty turned the ignition and the V8 roared into life, each cylinder popping with suppressed power. He then reversed and navigated his way out of the short-stay car park.

"Have to say, boss, you had a few people in Brissie dustin' off their dress uniforms. I bet when the funeral got cancelled there were plenty of managers who didn't know whether to cry or sing."

"What d'you mean?"

"The relief they avoided saying nice things about you must have been tempered by the return of their nemesis."

"Nemesis, eh? Them's big words, Scotty. You been reading books while I've been away?"

"Guess two weeks floating alone in a raft didn't cure your sarcasm."

"'Fraid not. I reckon it's hardwired into my DNA."

We were now motoring along Airport Drive, the lights of the city twinkling in the distance. I had the window down and the rush of air felt good on my face.

"So. You ever going to tell me the true story about your disappearance?"

I looked across at Scotty, who was staring out the windscreen, avoiding any eye contact. I paused before answering. "One day, mate, one day. You'll have to get me drunk, though, and I'll deny everything when I sober up. Let's say, my boating accident was media spin. You know how the government doesn't comment on operational matters regarding people smuggling."

He gave me a startled look. "People smuggling?"

"What? I didn't say that. Don't know what you're talking about, Scotty." I gripped his shoulder. "Just so you're aware, it turns out that along with the police, us ambos are bound by the Official Secrets Act."

"We are?"

"Apparently. Even if we're not, I don't want to be a test

case. They have enough shit on me that I could spend the rest of my life being some big dude's jail bitch."

"Holy fuck. It's almost worth driving you straight to a bottle shop to get you pissed."

"I'd love to, but not this trip. As you know, I've got to make good on some of the crap that went down last year."

"And I thought I was the shit magnet."

We drove on in silence while my mind jumped back to what had happened since the trawler sank. It felt like every conceivable government agency had interviewed me over three times, and eventually they decided a cover-up was the best outcome. At least that meant no one was sacked or reprimanded, but I was sure we'd all been blacklisted. I guess it was lucky that Miles and Charlie were happy on Mornington, and the last thing Gee and I wanted was promotion into a managerial role.

As to the refugees, the authorities were still looking for the first group, but if they found any, I was unlikely to hear. The second batch was now detained on the tiny Pacific island of Nauru, three thousand kilometres from the country they hoped to call home. Although their refugee status was being processed, they were out of sight, out of mind, and well away from any prying journalists. The only person to have come out on top was Rob. Due to the cover-up, his insurance claim was paid out almost immediately, and he ploughed his cash back into an even more expensive marlin boat.

Scotty looked uncomfortable as he asked another question. "So… is Amber still visiting, boss?"

I smiled. "Not so much now. Not the nightmares, anyway. I'm hoping this trip'll be part of the healing process."

He nodded. "Here's hoping."

After passing through the tunnels and emerging into the Central Business District, we wended our way through a maze of roads until we drew to a stop about twenty metres from a dim side street. I looked in disbelief at the darkened alleyway where I'd used Mr Wendal as bait to catch Boardie.

"You're shitting me, he's not still sleeping here is he?"

"Most nights since you asked me to check. Guess it's like a sacred site to him."

"Doubt it. He probably comes here wishing I let him die that night."

He shrugged. "Oh, those things you requested are on the back seat."

I reached behind me and grabbed them. "Cheers Scotty, wish me luck."

"If luck means you'll end up with Mr Wendal's stinking arse in my car, then forgive me if I don't."

I opened the door and stepped out. "Stop your whingin', I'll pay for a valet service if it makes you feel better."

"Add an external polish and you've got a deal."

I smiled at him and showed him my middle finger. "Polish this."

He grinned and returned the gesture as I walked off towards the alley. As in my dream, it was dark and foreboding, emanating the ever-present stench of garbage, but the bricks were warm to touch and there were no bats flying nearby. I sat down inside the entrance, so I was still within the glow of the streetlight, and flicked on the torch, sweeping the beam around until I found him.

His response was predictable. "Switch dat fuckin' ting out an' fuck off!"

I extinguished the light, but began tapping an enamel mug on the concrete. To my surprise, there were no more expletives, and after a pause, I could hear movement from within. Soon, Mr Wendal emerged from the shadows and sat cross-legged opposite me. We stared at one another for what seemed an age, but I knew it was not my place to speak first.

"I's wondered when yous'ud show up."

I nodded slowly and looked at my feet. "I've come to say sorry."

His rheumy eyes never wavered. "Dat may make yous feel better. But sayin' sorry don't do fuck all for me."

"Well, I'm sorry for what I did to you, Mr Gibson."

He blinked and his body stiffened, but then he relaxed back against the wall, all the time keeping his eyes on me. "Bin ages since anyones called me dat. Yous bin digging' up dirt on me, eh?"

"No, far from it. Over the last year I've made a good friend, Charlie Parker, who's another Lardil man. He told me your story, the real story. That bad stuff you think you did on Mornington? You didn't do it. You're innocent."

The stare continued until he rubbed his face and looked into his lap. "Don't know no fucka called Charlie Parker. Whys the fuck shoulda listen to anytin' yous says?"

I nodded. "I thought you might say that." As I handed him my phone, I hit the call button under the contact 'Naomi'. "Someone wants to speak to you. She's been searching for you for years. She never gave up hope."

He rolled his head to one side as his brow wrinkled, but he took the phone and held it to his ear. A second later his eyes closed, shoulders sagged, and he rested his head back on the wall. "Mam."

I'm not sure who was the first to cry, but my vision was blurred as I saw tears rolling down his craggy cheeks and he let out a deep sigh.

They spoke for a while before he returned my phone and wiped his face. This time I was the one who broke the silence. "Our flights are booked for tomorrow, and tonight we're staying in a hotel. Gotta get you spruced up for your homecoming. Those are your mother's orders and she's a lady no one should mess with. Believe me, I know."

He rubbed his nose and looked me up and down before retrieving his own battered enamel mug from his bag. "Did ya just bring dat cup to knock on the ground, or are we's gonna share some of dat grog ya got der... brudda?"

I grinned at him and gave him a nod before reaching for the box of wine.

ACKNOWLEDGMENTS

Back in 2014, I somehow managed to write the initial draft of *Beneath Contempt* in about five months. Since then, other than receiving the initial feedback, the manuscript languished in the recesses of my computer until I plucked up the courage to publish *Dead Regular*. When I wrote at the end of 2020 that the sequel was coming soon, I mistakenly thought I'd completed most of the corrections. But the fact that it has taken almost a year to get the book up to scratch is testament to the dedication of my editing team, who have often read my work multiple times for no other reason than their faith in me as a writer. Therefore I would like to thank Lynnette Cameron, Amie Cawood, Damien Storeywood, Gaye Franks, Glenn Davies, John Bathurst and Lisa King for their work on the initial draft and Petra Johnson, Qbone Kenobe, Vicki Nelson and Jack Roney for the detailed feedback they provided through the BetaBooks system.

For the record, I have worked on numerous tropical islands in my former life as a marine biologist, but I am yet to visit any in the Gulf of Carpentaria. Therefore, other than online research, my knowledge of Mornington Island was gleaned through interviewing two paramedics who worked there for three years. I am most grateful to Larry & Lynette Nardello, who gave me a wonderful insight into their experiences and I used their stories to form the basis of Jono's on-island escapades. Although I thought it would be disingenuous to avoid the plight of First Nation's people in *Dead Regular*, I did feel guilty for using an overused stereotype in the form of Mr Wendal. I hope I have made amends in this book with Charlie, one of my favourite characters, and thank both Metesha Cox and Dawn Aaskov for their feedback from a First Nation's perspective.

And once again, saving the most important to last, I would like to thank my ever-supportive mother and my wonderful wife. The latter informed me she hoped I'd be more 'gushing' in this acknowledgement than the last. Unfortunately for her, I'm someone who finds it difficult to gush, so I'm hoping that the dedication will suffice.

Many thanks to all those who have helped get this book into the hands of readers.

ABOUT THE AUTHOR

Harry Colfer is the pseudonym of a critical care paramedic who lives and works in Brisbane, Australia. Although his stories are totally fictional, his writing style is very realistic and he maintains a healthy level of paranoia with respect to his anonymity.

To date he has published twenty-two short stories in the *Ambo Tales From The Frontline* series and plans to write another ten, one for each of the thirty-two AMPDS codes, the system used worldwide to categorise emergency calls.

He is currently writing the third novel in the Jono series, *High Acuity*, with the fourth and final book existing only as ideas, notes, and a title, *Show Cause*.

WWW.HARRYCOLFER.COM

facebook.com/harry.colfer.1
twitter.com/Harry_Colfer
instagram.com/harrycolfer
amazon.com/author/harrycolfer

Printed in Great Britain
by Amazon

70023081R00199